CHRONIC PANCREATITIS

Edited by **David Sutherland**

Chronic Pancreatitis
Edited by David Sutherland

Published by InTech
Janeza Trdine 9, 51000 Rijeka, Croatia

Publishing Process Manager Vedran Greblo

Technical Editor Teodora Smiljanic

Cover Designer InTech Design Team

Additional hard copies can be obtained from orders@intechopen.com

Chronic Pancreatitis, Edited by David Sutherland
p. cm.
ISBN 978-953-51-0011-9

For EU product safety concerns:
IN TECH d.o.o., Prolaz Marije Krucifikse Kozulić 3, 51000 Rijeka, Croatia,
info@intechopen.com or visit our website at intechopen.com.

Meet the editor

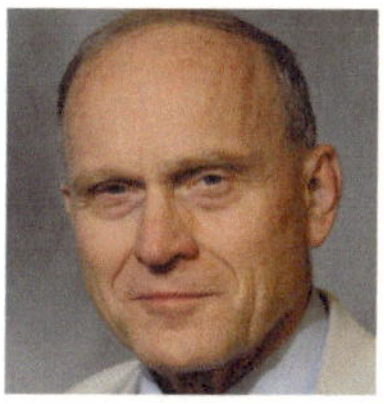

Dr David Sutherland graduated from the University of Minnesota (UM) Medical School in 1966. In Medical School he started his research career in immunology, and made seminal contributions on the role of gut-associated lymphoid tissue in the development of the immune response. After 2 years in the Army, he completed a Surgery Residency at the UM in 1975, a Transplant Fellowship in 1976, and then joined the faculty. He received his Ph.D. in 1977, was promoted to Professor of Surgery in 1984, founded and is Director of the UM Diabetes Institute for Immunology and Transplantation since 1994, was Head of the Division of Transplantation from 1995 to 2009, and has been holder of a Diabetes Research Chair since 2003. Dr. Sutherland is an author on over 1500 publications. His academic interests are wide, with special emphasis on beta cell replacement therapy for diabetes mellitus (which led to the development of interest in chronic pancreatitis and treatment by total pancreatectomy and auto islet transplantation); immunosuppression management; and on training clinical/basic scientists in translational research. He began clinical islet transplants at the UM in 1974 (the first in the world). Since 1978 he has been director of the UM pancreas transplant program, the oldest (began in 1966) and largest (more than 2000 cases done since he took charge) in the world. He founded the International Pancreas Transplant Registry in 1980. More than 100 physicians who trained with Dr. Sutherland developed or now direct pancreas/ islet transplant programs around the world, including in-treatment of chronic pancreatitis. He is Past-President of the American Society of Transplant Surgeons (1990-91), The Cell Transplant Society (1995-96), the International Society for Pancreas and Islet Transplantation (1996-97) and The Transplantation Society (2002-2004). He has served on the editorial boards of many journals, including Cell Transplantation, Diabetes, Transplantation, Transplantation Proceedings, and Pancreas. He has been Editor-in-Chief for Clinical Transplantation since January, 2007. Though diverse but related, his main interest currently remains in the treatment of chronic pancreatitis.

Contents

Preface

Chronic pancreatitis is a disease of diverse etiologies in which the main problem is pain. The pain can be devastating, lead to narcotic dependence, severely impair quality of life and may require surgery in an attempt to alleviate pain. Pain in chronic pancreatitis may be due to increased intraductal pressure secondary to partial complete blockage of the duct, or it may be intrinsic to the diseased gland that itself from the inflammatory changes or the sequelae thereof. It remains a challenge to physicians and surgeons in regard to treatment.

This book addresses many issues of chronic pancreatitis and it is divided into two sections: basic science investigations in animal models of chronic pancreatitis and a clinical section on the diagnosis and treatment of chronic pancreatitis. It should be noted that chronic pancreatitis initially affects the exocrine portion of the gland, but secondary involvement of the islets of Langerhans can result in the diabetes mellitus. The principle of treatment is to preserve as much pancreatic function as possible while alleviating the pain, again a challenge to surgeons and a stimulus to develop nonsurgical treatments to mitigate the inflammation and fibrosis of chronic pancreatitis.

In this book there are three basic science contributions. The first, by Hong Bin Liu in Nankai Clinical College of Tianjin Medical University, includes a comprehensive review of the pathology of chronic pancreatitis and then, in a rat model, summarizes the data demonstrating that bone marrow-derived stem cells may be recruited directly to the organ and contribute to amelioration of chronic pancreatitis. The MSC recruit and reside in an injured pancreas as C cells and from there they differentiate into pancreatic target cells or functional cells such as acinar cells, islet cells, ductal cells, and pancreatic stem cells. The regenerating effects to the paracrine autocrine function, secreting many active molecules such as stem cell growth factor that antagonize the effects of pearl inflammatory cytokines, alleviate the pathological injury. Indices have already been used clinically to treat patients with certain metabolic diseases as well as for other use. Thus the development of MSC therapy for chronic pancreatitis especially if able to reply early, shows great promise.

Chronic pancreatitis is a progressive fibro-inflammatory disorder characterized pathologically by fibrosis and permanent destruction of acinar cells. Regardless of the etiology and histological, pictures are fairly similar. The islets of Langerhans are generally preserved until chronic pancreatitis is advanced, but pancreatic diabetes is not uncommon. In studies by Karin Westlund from the University of Kentucky Medical Center, a separate approach of using gene therapy for HSV-Enkephalin to reduce fibrosis inflammation and pain is used. In her studies she was able to test pain sensitivity for rats with or without pancreatitis. The pro Enkephalin gene in the pancreas was repaired and significantly reduced pain-related behaviors in rodent pancreatitis models. Thus, the gene therapeutic approach that promotes the endogenous OP8 Enkephalin is clearly delivered by the neuronal system and has clinical relevance for reducing inflammation induced pain related behavior and tissue destruction. The gene therapy approach was used to over express the precursor of the endogenous opiate peptide metenkephalin and was found to induce histological and behavioral changes. Thus this approach also has great promise for clinical application.

The third basic science contribution is by Garofita-Olivia Mateescu and associates in Bucharest, Romania. This group studied the pancreatic acinar and island neogenesis in relationship to vascular and matrix dynamics. These studies have great relevance to prevention of diabetes in chronic pancreatitis via stellite cells. This group found that multiple factors were important in that pathogenesis of chronic pancreatitis that lead to parenchymal destruction and fibrosis but also with elements of acino-insular neogenesis. They noted endocrine parenchymal regeneration in histopathological human pancreatitis specimens and animal models in the study of a wide variety of pathological processes, including human satellite cells connective with central regulator cell and pancreatic fibrosis and they found differences according to etiology. In immunochemical results in the dynamics, acino-island neogenesis did not totally clarify the subject, partly explained in the human model subjects exposed to many factors in different evolutionary stages while in the animals those factors can be controlled. Most important was the identification of endocrine parenchymal regeneration issues. The authors show the potential to preserve both pancreatic exocrine and endocrine function in chronic pancreatitis.

The clinical section is led by a chapter by José Ardengh and Eder Rios Lima-Filho, "The Role of Endoscopic Ultrasound to Diagnose, Exclude or Establish the Parenquimal Changes in Chronic Pancreatitis". Again, because chronic pancreatitis is an inflammatory disease with progressive and, in their view, irreversible morphological changes, endoscopic ultrasound is valuable in the diagnosis in staging the disease. However, it should be noted that the endoscopic ultrasound which identifies 9 criteria, chronic pancreatitis can be associated with as few as 1, but if 6 are present, chronic pancreatitis is almost always present histologically. However, having less than 6 does not rule out pancreatitis. This group shows the sensitivity and specificity of the EUS as compared to other studies such as retrograde cholangiopancreatography and also compared to magnetic resonance cholangiopancreatography. Correlations were made and discordance was found. This chapter points out the advantages and pitfalls of EUS in the diagnosis of chronic pancreatitis. Thus EUS is proving to be of value to diagnose chronic pancreatitis and its complications. It has to be interpreted in the light of other studies of the pancreas and as pointed out by the authors, it is not yet the gold standard if indeed there is any good standard for diagnosis of chronic pancreatitis. Minimal change chronic pancreatitis is a real entity associated with pain, particularly in young women, and may be missed entirely by EUS.

Chapter five is written by Yue Sun Cheung and Paul Bo-San Lai at the Chinese University of Hong Kong and they have focused on endoscopic treatment in chronic pancreatitis. Thus, extraction of intraductal stones or chronic pancreatitis that may be associated with sphincter of Oddi dysfunction, can now be treated by the endoscopic approach and it is a matter of the probability of pain relief. Pancreatic sphincterotomy and stenting of the pancreatic duct in addition to stone extraction in ultrasound-guided pseudocyst drainage and celiac plexus blocks are addressed. The response rate in endoscopic treatment of chronic pancreatitis is quite variable and there are a significant number of failures which then can come to surgery.

Surgical options for chronic pancreatitis are presented by Fazl Q. Parray of Kashmir India with the principle of trying to preserve as much function as possible while relieving the pain is the main focus. It is a very good historical review and even the origin of the anatomy of the pancreas and identification of disease. This chapter is extremely comprehensive, reviewing more than 20 surgical procedures, including duct drainage procedures, partially ablative procedures, and totally ablative. He shows that both resection of the pancreas and drainage, when combined, can give good results but that pain relief with total pancreatectomy is somewhat higher. In this chapter, chronic pancreatitis is also reviewed as far as the inflammatory and fibrosis process and how these aspects relate to relief of pain.

The final chapter is the role of total pancreatectomy and islet autotransplant for chronic pancreatitis. This approach completely removes the causes of pain. However, pain may continue for patients that have been on long-term narcotics and had long-term pain from opiate induced hyperalgesia or from central sensitization of pain. Nevertheless, pain relief achieved appears higher than with other procedures taking into account the different populations that may occur in each. Total pancreatectomy by itself is the antithesis to preserve as much function as possible, but with islet autotransplant at least beta cell function is preserved. More than 90% of the patients are C-peptide positive after the total pancreatectomy and islet autotransplant and more than 80% have a normal glycosolated hemoglobin. About a third of the patients are insulin-independent. Thus, islet autotransplantation is highly successful in the setting of total pancreatectomy and should certainly be considered as a front line surgical procedure in those who fail endoscopic duct drainage procedures.

In summary, chronic pancreatitis is a complex disease with various etiologies of pathogenesis, but characterized by fibrosis and inflammation in the pancreas, some of which cannot be detected by imaging studies because of the minimal changes that can be associated with severe pain. Treatment options are discussed include using stem cells and gene therapy with HSV-Enkephalin. Such treatments currently would be clinically feasible. Finally the diagnosis and treatment of chronic pancreatitis is covered in the clinical chapters with many approaches indicating that not one glove fits all. Chronic pancreatitis remains a clinical challenge for alleviation of pain, reduction of narcotics, and to improve quality of life. All of the chapters in this book are forward-looking and relevant for treatment of tomorrow's, if not today's, patients.

Prof. David Sutherland,
University of Minnesota,
USA

Part 1

Basic Science Issues in Chronic Pancreatitis

1

Bone Marrow Derived Mesenchymal Stem Cells Are Recruited into Injured Pancreas and Contribute to Amelioration of the Chronic Pancreatitis in Rats

Hong Bin Liu
Department of Pharmacology, Tianjin Institute of Acute Abdominal Diseases, Nankai Clinical College of Tianjin Medical University, China

1. Introduction

Chronic pancreatitis is characterized by destruction of pancreatic parenchyma, inflammatory cell infiltration, and irregular fibrosis, accompanied by insufficient pancreatic exocrine, endocrine function and clinically by chronic abdominal pain, diabetes, maldigestion, malnutrition and even pancreatic cancer.The proposed pancreas regeneration mechanisms have included ductal progenitors, acinar transdifferentiation, circulating progenitors, and putative pancreatic stem cells (Granger and Kushner, 2009; Pittenger et al., 2009). Bone marrow (BM) harbors a pool of stem cells capable of differentiating into multiple tissue types. Bone marrow-derived cells have the potential to transdifferentiate into multiple lineage cells. With their regenerative potential and immunoregulatory effect, MSC therapy is a promising tool in the treatment of degenerative, inflammatory, and autoimmune diseases, including chronic pancreatitis.

2. Histopathology of chronic pancreatitis

Chronic pancreatitis (CP) is a progressive fibroinflammatory disorder of the pancreas characterized pathologically by fibrosis and permanent destruction of acinar cells. Although the etiologies of CP may differ, the histologic features of the disease are similar. The key histopathologic features of CP are pancreatic fibrosis, acinar atrophy, chronic inflammation, and distorted and blocked ducts. In sequential fashion, variable interlobular, lobular, and ductal fibrosis may be seen throughout the gland in the early stages of CP and become more diffuse as the disease progresses. As acinar cells within the lobules are destroyed by fibrosis, exocrine dysfunction ensues. The islets of Langerhans are generally preserved until CP is advanced, and endocrine dysfunction generally lags behind that of the exocrine pancreas. In advanced stages, subintimal fibrosis of blood vessels can be demonstrated and nerve fibers are drawn into the fibrotic process. Infiltrating into these areas of fibrosis are lymphocytes, plasma cells, and macrophages.

Pancreatic stellate cells (PSCs) play a key role in pancreatic fibrosis. The PSC has been demonstrated in vitro and in vivo to be primarily involved with collagen deposition and eventual fibrosis. PSCs are activated by cytokines released from infiltrating leucocytes and the injured acinar cells. The end stage of chronic pancreatitis is identified by loss of all secretory tissue, disappearance of inflammatory cells, and intense fibrosis. This progression resembles that from chronic active hepatitis to liver cirrhosis. Additional distinctive histologic features have been described in some forms of CP, such as extensive pancreatic calcification in tropical pancreatitis and a prominent lymphocytic and plasma cell infiltrate in autoimmune pancreatitis.

3. The mechanisms of pancreas self-renew

How does the injured pancreas self-renew ? Where do the cells involving the pancreatic regeneration and self-renewing come from? These are the questions have not been clarified for a long time. Pancreas regeneration has been studied for more than 30 years and until now, the search for specific pancreatic stem cells has focused on pancreatic ductular cells, pre-existing β cells, and embryonic stem cells.

Pancreatic ductal cell lines and primary ductal cells have been successfully differentiated into insulin-expressing cells by in vitro approaches, including treatment with growth factors (e.g., EGF, Gastrin, exendin), expression of pancreatic transcription factors, and aggregation (Xia et al, 2009; Hanley et al, 2008; Weir et al, 2000,2002,2009). Neogenesis of insulin-producing cells from differentiated pancreatic ductal cells results from their dedifferentiation into progenitors, expressing markers like PDX1 (Pancreatic and duodenal homeobox 1), which redifferentiate into insulin-producing and other pancreatic cells. Hence, "terminally"differentiated ductal cells can be considered facultative stem cells. Like ductal cells, lineage-marked acinar cells in response to EGF underwent in vitro differentiation into insulin expressing cells (Minami et al.,2005). A role for acinar-to-ductal transdifferentiation has also been suggested in conversion of acinar cells into endocrine cells. These observations demonstrate that multiple cell sources can differentiate into insulin-producing cells under in vitro culture conditions.

Animal models in which pancreatic endocrine and exocrine regeneration can be observed include chemically induced models of pancreatic injury following administration of alloxan (Davidson et al.,1989; Waguri et al.,1997), streptozotocin (Like & Rossini, 1976) or caerulein (Elsasser et al., 1986), dietary copper deprivation (Abdullah et al.,2000), physical disruption of pancreatic duct function by cellophane wrapping of the organ (Wolf-Coote et al., 1996; Rafaeloff et al., 1997)or ligation of the pancreatic duct, hemipancreatectomy (Weir et al.,1993; Sharma et al., 1999) and local over-expression of Reg1 (Yamaoka et al., 2000), IFNγ (Kritzik et al.,1999; Gu et al., 1997) or TGF-α (Sandgren et al., 1990). Although the triggers may differ, in each of these models pancreatic regeneration is thought to occur through the expansion of progenitor cells present either in, or closely associatedwith, the ductal epithelium. In these models, both endocrine and exocrine cells have been observed to arise from duct cells. Supporting this observation, 'transitional' cells have been identified that co-express ductal markers with endocrine or exocrine cell-specific markers, suggesting a reprogramming of duct-like cells (Gu et al., 1993,1994; Wang et al.,1995).

In many of these models of regeneration, there is a striking proliferation of ductal epithelia and newly formed ductal complexes. In the 90% pancreatectomy model, regeneration has been suggested to mimic embryonic pancreogenesis with proliferation occurring initially from expansion of the common pancreatic duct epithelium followed by branching of smaller ductules and subsequent regeneration of exocrine, endocrine and mature duct cells (Weir et al.,1993). In contrast, in models of exocrine pancreatic injury, ductal proliferation has been ascribed to condensation of the existing ductular network (Kelly et al.,1999), de-differentiation of acinar cells to duct-like cells, or, as in the pancreatectomy model, to proliferation of the ductal epithelia. In summary, models of pancreas regeneration reveal that islet and acinar regeneration occur proximate to ductal tissue.

Acinar and endocrine cells probably have a similar epigenetic profile as they share a common multipotent progenitor, which should make transdifferentiation of acinar cells into β-cells easier than from non-pancreatic cells (Gu et al.,2003).

In the adult pancreas, acinar cell growth is influenced by hormonal stimulation, notably by the gut hormone cholecystokinin (CCK). It is reported that CCK induces adaptive acinar cell growth by causing nuclear translocation of nuclear factor of activated Tcells (NFAT) via the Ca^{2+}/calmodulin-dependent phosphatase calcineurin (Gurda et al.,2008). In response to injury, the pancreas activates regenerative processes to maintain tissue homeostasis. The prevailing notion is that after injury, acinar cells might dedifferentiate into a ductal epithelium that expresses early developmental factors. These 'facultative progenitor cells' would then redifferentiate into mature acinar cells. Two recent reports highlight the importance of the expression of embryonic factors by acinar cells in guiding the regenerative process. It is showed that reactivation of the Notch signaling pathway during injury from caerulein-induced pancreatitis is required for acinar cell regeneration (Siveke et al., 2008). Fendrich et al. found that embryonic signaling by Hedgehog was upregulated in acinar cells after caerulein-induced pancreatitis, and that its blockade either pharmacologically or genetically, using PDX1 or elastase-Cre recombinase, allowed the formation of a ductal epithelium from acinar cells, but it did not permit the redifferentiation into acini (Fendrich et al., 2008). Intriguingly, the authors suggest that the 'redifferentiation arrest' might provide a link between pancreatitis injury and subsequent neoplasia. The results also underscore the capacity of the acinar cell to revert to an earlier progenitor state in response to injury.

Recent findings suggest that pancreatic progenitor cells might not be limited to the pancreas, but that cells from other tissues could be mobilized and induced to differentiate and contribute to the regenerative process. Stimuli such as surgical removal of a part of the pancreas, cellophane wrapping and transplantation of bone marrow cells can induce pancreatic regeneration to different extents.

Advances in defining the molecular basis of early pancreogenesis have contributed to an understanding of the process of regeneration that occurs in animal models of pancreatic injury and diabetes. However, pancreatic progenitor cell populations remain poorly defined and the subject of considerable debate (Andrew et al., 2004).

The question remains open whether a pluripotent pancreatic progenitor cell exists or whether duct associated regeneration reflects the inherent plasticity of these cells. GLUT-2 (glucose transporter 2) has been reported to be a potential marker of progenitor cells because it is induced in ductal or islet cells in models of regeneration.

In suspension culture, rat acini lose their exocrine phenotype and express the duct-cell markers cytokeratin (CK)-7 and CK-20 coincident with PDX1, Ptf1a and Flk1. The continued expression of Ptf1a and the induction of PDX1 and Flk1 in these cells is particularly intriguing given that both PDX1 and Ptf1a are markers of early pancreatic progenitors and that the ligand of Flk1, VEGF has been implicated in early pancreogenesis and endocrine development. The induced expression of genes such as PDX1, GLUT-2, Flk1 and Kuz during pancreas regeneration is particularly interesting as it is clearly reminiscent of embryonic gene expression programs. This recapitulation of embryonic phenotype is a common theme in many of the animal models of regeneration and is indicative of the presence of progenitor cells in the adult pancreas (O'Reilly et al., 1997; Song et al., 1999).

An important feature of epithelial cells is their ability to continuously regenerate. This process, in the adult, is limited to different degrees in different epithelial organs by the rate of cell division. For example, epidermal keratinocytes and intestinal cells have a rapid turnover, whereas pancreatic epithelial cells replicate slowly.

The existence of organ-specific adult stem cells is now widely accepted. However, it is clear that somatic adult stem cells are rare and therefore difficult to isolate and study. They reside in a microenvironment or niche (Schofield et al., 1978), within which they are closely associated with tissue stromal cells and daughter cells, which controls and determines their fate. Identifying the presumptive pancreatic stem cell niche and defining the cellular and molecular components that regulate pancreas specific developmental programmes remains the subject of intensive research.

4. Properties and immunosuppressive activity of MSCs

Mesenchymal stem cells (MSCs) are non-hematopoietic cells with multi-lineage potential (Barry &Murphy,2004). They have been shown to differentiate into various tissues of mesodermal origin, such as adipocytes, osteoblasts, chondrocytes, tenocytes, and skeletal myocytes. They can be isolated from bone marrow (BM) and various other sources such as umbilical cord blood or adipose tissues and have the capacity to extensively proliferate in vitro. Their capacity to differentiate into various lineages and their in vitro proliferative potential makes them attractive targets for regenerative medicine applications.

It has been demonstrated that MSCs possess immunomodulatory properties. MSCs are shown to inhibit T cell proliferation and to influence the maturation and expression profile of professional antigen presenting cells such as dendritic cells (DCs). For instance, MSCs from various species (humans, rodents and primates) can suppress the response of T cells to mitogenic and polyclonal stimuli and to their cognate peptide. Such an effect is not cognate dependent because it can still be observed using MSCs from third-party donors fully mismatched for the MHC haplotype of the responder T cells or MSCs which are constitutively negative for MHC molecule expression. MSC-induced unresponsiveness lacks any selectivity, as it similarly affects memory and naïve T cells as well as $CD4^+$ and $CD8^+$ subsets.

The characterisation of MSC-induced anergic T cells showed that the inhibitory effect of MSCs is directed mainly at the level of T cell proliferation. T cells stimulated in the presence of MSCs are arrested at the G1 phase as a result of cyclin D2 downregulation. The expression of CD25 and CD69 markers of T cell activation is completely unaffected by MSC co-culture, and inhibition of T cell effector functions can be reversed by MSCs removal. Whilst MSCs induce an unresponsive T cell profile, they can prevent the apoptosis of activated T cells, indicating that MSC-mediated immunosuppression results from an induced division arrest anergy.

The effects of MSCs on immune responses are not confined to T cells. Although they are susceptible to recognition and lysis by IL-2 activated cells and natural killer (NK) cells in vitro, due to their low expression of HLA class I, MSCs have been demonstrated to be capable of inhibiting the proliferation of interleukin-2 (IL-2) or IL-15 stimulated NK cells. Whilst there is agreement on the immunosuppressive ability of MSCs on NK cells, their influence on NK cell-mediated cytotoxicity remains controversial. Initial data suggested that MSCs could inhibit the cytolytic activity of IL-2 activated NK cells, but more recent studies have shown that lysis of HLA I positive allogeneic targets by freshly isolated NK cells is not inhibited by MSCs. NK cells' cytokine production is also influenced by MSCs, which are able to induce the release of IFN-γand TNF-α.

The effect of MSCs on B cell proliferation remains controversial. Studies in the mouse and humans showed that MSCs inhibit B cell proliferation, inducing a block in G0/G1 phase of the cell cycle. MSCs have also been shown to inhibit the differentiation of B cells to antibody secreting cells as well as downregulating CXCR4, CXCR5 and CCR7 chemokine receptors. In contrast, other studies have suggested that human MSCs promote the proliferation and differentiation of B cells from healthy donors and patients with systemic lupus erythematosus. Although apparently in contradiction, the opposing results of these studies can be reconciled by the different conditions in which B cells have been stimulated. As a result of different B cell stimulation, the secreted cytokines could in fact polarise MSC towards a proinflammatory phenotype. This concept is well established for other cell types with regulatory functions, such as monocytes/macrophages.

Considering their regenerative potential and immunoregulatory effect, MSC-therapy is a promising tool in the treatment of degenerative, inflammatory, and autoimmune diseases. However, the current understanding from results of clinical trials is that MSC-therapy is safe but its therapeutic efficiency needs to be improved (Trento & Dazzi, 2010).

5. Experimental study of MSCs on chronic pancreatitis

One additional and crucial feature of MSCs is their ability to selectively migrate to sites of injury. However, the use of MSCs in pancreatic regeneration is just now emerging.

With above-mentioned provocative in vitro and in vivo observations, we sought to observe the protective properties and to explore the potential mechanism of the BMSCs in treating CP rat model. Our study demonstrated that BMSCs in rats caused (1) an intensified and much higher GFP (green fluorescent proteins) fluorescence expression of positive GFP-labeled cells in the pancreatic tissue of model plus BMSCs (GFP^+) group compared with that of the control group (Fig 3) ; (2) a marked attenuation of pancreatic pathological injury and fibrosis of BMSCs treated group compared to those of model group (Fig 2; Fig 4; Table 1) ;(3) a significant reduction of pancreatic CTGF, TGF-β, type-I collagen, type-III collagen and MPO activities(Table 2). Our findings suggest that BMSCs have obvious therapeutic effects in the treatment of CP, which may be related to their recruitments to the damaged pancreatic tissue as seeds cells and their inhibition of CTGF,TGF-β release by autocrine or paracrine effects, thus decreasing the type-I collagen, type-III collagen and MPO producing.

In our study, it was revealed that BMSCs only recruited to the injured pancreas. In the sham plus BMSCs (GFP+) group, although BMSCs (GFP+) were transplanted to the rats as model plus BMSCs (GFP+) group, the GFP fluorescence was still absent in the pancreas tissue(Fig 3). As for the mechanism of BMSCs homing to the injured pancreas, a growing number of studies of various pathologic conditions have demonstrated that MSC selectively home to sites of injury, irrespective of the tissue. Homing involves a cascade of processes initiated by shear resistant adhesive interactions between flowing cells and the vascular endothelium at target tissue. This process is mediated by 'homing receptors' expressed on circulating cells that engage relevant endothelial co-receptors, resulting in cell-tethering and rolling contacts on the endothelial surface. This is typically followed by chemokine triggered activation of integrin adhesiveness, firm adhesion and extravasation.

Therefore, we may deduce the mechanisms of MSCs treating CP as followed three points. The first one is that MSCs can recruit to and reside in the injured pancreas as the "seed cells", also they can differentiate into the pancreatic "target cells" or "functional cells" such as acinar cells, Islet(like) cells, ductal cells and pancreatic stem cells, etc. Second, MSCs exert their regenerating effects through the paracrine/autocrine function, secreting many kinds of bioactive molecules (such as stem cell growth factor, SCGF), antagonizing the effects of proinflammatory cytokines, alleviating the pathological injury, inhibiting the proliferation of the pancreatic stellate cells. The latter is that MSCs can ameliorate the immune-inflammatory injury within the pancreas by their immunosuppressive and immunoregulatory functions which include inhibiting the T lymphocytes, cyto-toxic T lymphocytes, NK cells, macrophages and mast cells. However, the details of the mechanisms abovementioned remain an active area of investigation.

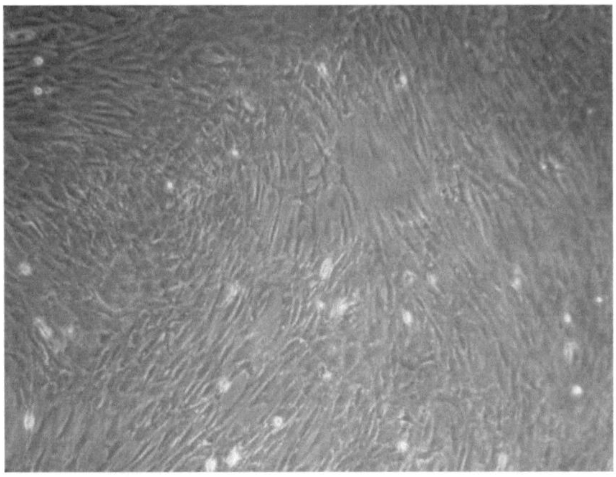

Fig. 1. Subcultured BMSCs in vitro. Phase contrast micrograph of mesenchymal stem cells cultured on day seven passage 2 (40×). Rat BMSCs were successfully isolated from bone marrow via gradient centrifugation, expanded in monolayer culture. Most of the non-adherent cells were removed during the first media change at 24 h. Three days after culture, the BMSCs began to stretch. Colonies of fibroblast-like cells attached to the plastic were evident at day 4–5 after initial seeding. Cell colonies were formed and number of adherent cells increased rapidly, BMSCs reached 80-90% of confluence by 12 day and arranged regularly in the swirl shape.

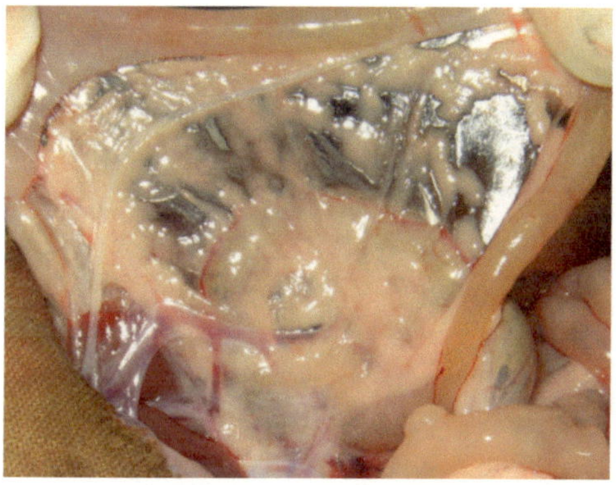

(a) Sham plus BMSCs (GFP^{+})

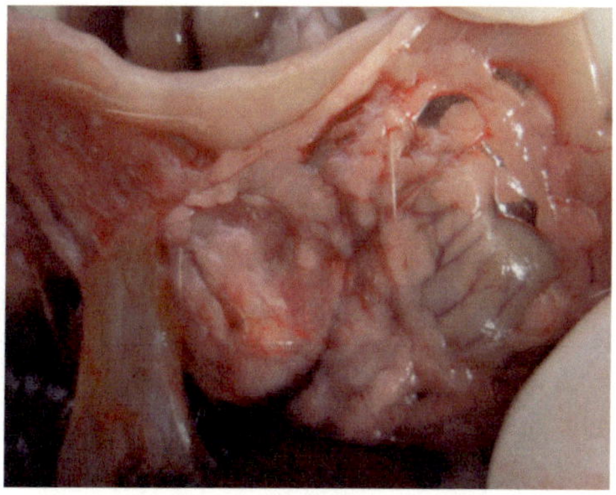

(b) Chronic pancreatitis model

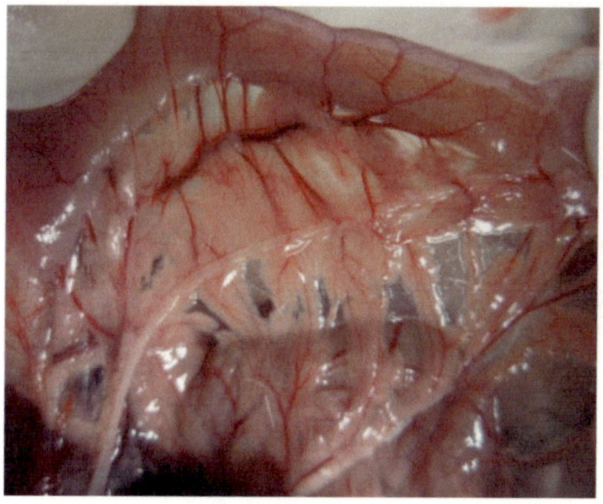

(c) Model plus BMSCs(GFP+)

Fig. 2. Gross appearance of pancreas tissue in sham plus BMSCs (GFP^{+}) (a), model (b) and model plus BMSCs (GFP^{+}) groups (c). a and c, pancreas has an intact appearance. b, note the scattered thickening, swelling foci and markedly dilated biliopancreatic duct.

	n	Histologic score	Fibrosis score
sham+BMSCs (GFP^{+})	10	0	0
model	10	7.92±2.58*	1.98±0.57*
model+BMSCs (GFP^{+})	10	2.17±0.37#	0.38±0.09#

*P < 0.001 vs sham +BMSCs (GFP^{+}) group. #†P <0.01 vs model group

Table 1. Histopathologic and fibrosis scores of pancreas tissue in all groups (mean±SD)

(a) Sham plus BMSCs (GFP+)

(b) Chronic pancreatitis mode

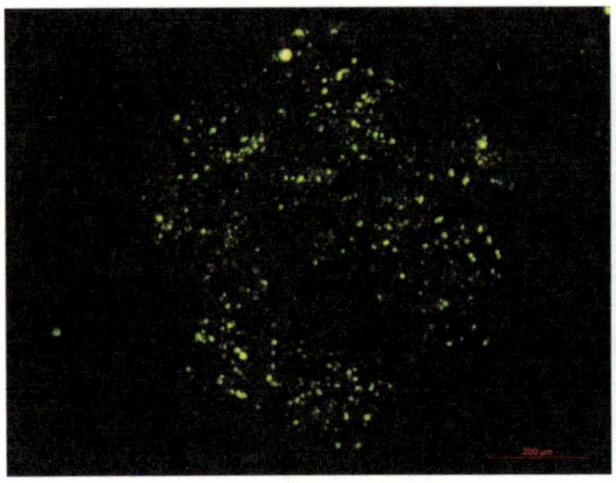

(c) Model plus BMSCs(GFP+)
(low magnification)

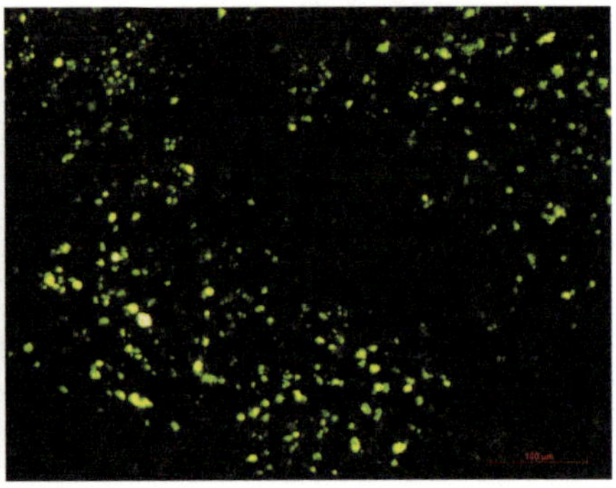

(d) Model plus BMSCs(GFP+)
(medium magnification)

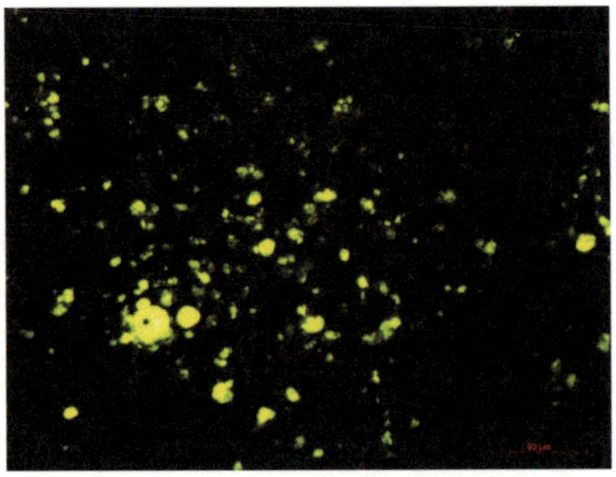

(e) Model plus BMSCs(GFP^{+})
(high magnification)

Fig. 3. GFP^{+}-BMSCs in the frozen pancreatic sections. No positive green fluorescence appeared in the pancreatic sections of sham plus BMSCs (GFP^{+}) group (a), model (b).GFP signals were clearly observed in pancreas from frozen sections after GFP^{+}-BMSCs transplantation of model plus BMSCs (GFP^{+}) group examined in fluorescence microscopy(c, low magnification; d, medium magnification; e, high magnification).

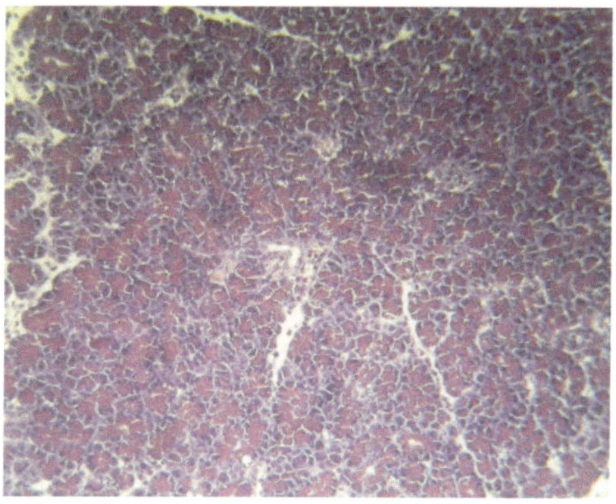

(a) Sham plus BMSCs (GFP+)

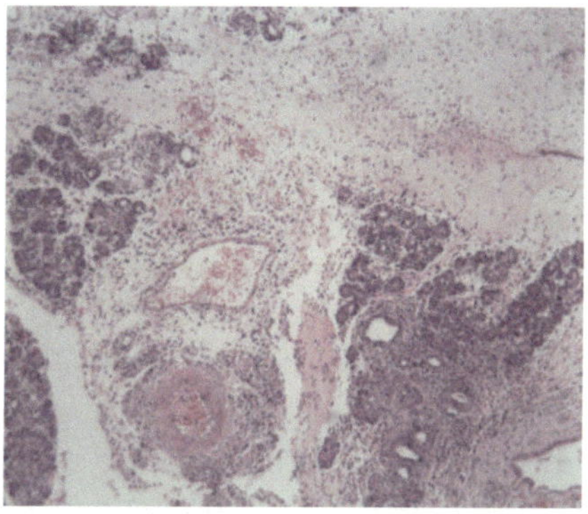

(b) Chronic pancreatitis mode

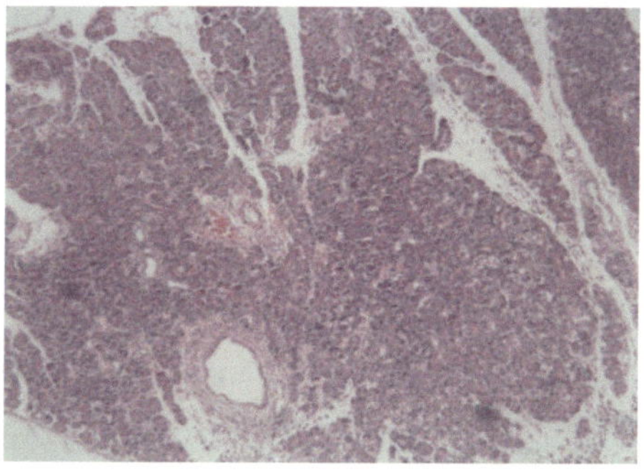

(c) Model plus BMSCs(GFP+)

Fig. 4. Representative light microscopic appearances of the pancreas stained with hematoxylin and eosin (H&E). a. In sham plus BMSCs (GFP+) group, no alteration was observed. b. In model group, massive infiltration of inflammatory cells, with disappearance of acinar cells are evident. c. In model plus BMSCs (GFP+) group, the distribution of fibrosis and inflammatory cells were markedly attenuated and acinar cells and lobular architecture can be seen.

	n	CTGF (pg/ mg prot)	TGF-β (pg/ mg prot)	collagen I (pg/ mg prot)	collagen III (ng/ mg prot)	MPO (mU/mg prot)
sham+BMSCs (GFP+)	10	19.8±9.8	10.1±2.9	60.9±15.1	18.4±6.2	0.41±0.14
model	10	279.8±20.8*	58.7±9.1*	245.7±35.8*	73.1±10.4*	2.75±0.47
model+BMSCs (GFP+)	10	121.4±20.1#	18.9±4.7#	142.9±28.5#	35.8±10.1#	1.12±0.18

*P < 0.001 vs sham +BMSCs (GFP+) group. #†P <0.01 vs model group

Table 2. Pancreatic CTGF, TGF-β, collagen I, collagen III and MPO contents in all groups (mean±SD)

6. Safety issues

The first clinical trials with adult stem/progenitor cells to repair non-haematopoietic tissues were carried out with MSCs (Prockop et al., 2007). The initial clinical trials with MSCs were in osteogenesis imperfecta patients (Horwitz et al.,2001) and in patients suffering mucopolysaccharidoses (Koc et al.,2002). Other indications for which clinical trials using MSCs have been initiated are suppression of GVHD severe autoimmune diseases, repair of skeletal tissue, amyotrophic lateral sclerosis, chronic spinal cord injury, non-healing chronic wounds, vascular disease, coronary artery disease and myocardial infarction. Currently, the largest number of clinical trials is in patients with heart disease with MSCs.

As of this writing, more than 100 clinical trials involving MSCs transplantation have been registered with the US Food and Drug Administration (www.clinicaltrials.gov). While most of the studies are currently ongoing or are small Phase I and Phase II safety trials, current findings suggest that MSCs transplants are safe and offer no suggestion of malignancy risk.

Currently, bone marrow, subcutaneous adipose tissue and umbilical cord blood are among the main sources for isolating MSCs. Human trials of MSCs transplantation are roughly evenly divided between the use of autologous and allogeneic cells and these trials employ both freshly-isolated and ex-vivo culture expanded cell populations. While most MSCs used for transplant are derived from BM, cells isolated from adipose, umbilical cord, and other MSC sources such as peripheral blood liver are being employed. These clinical trials employ MSCs for a multitude of different purposes in different disease states, including tissue replacement in musculoskeletal, cardiac and liver diseases, and as immunomodulatory cells to mitigate GVHD, organ transplant rejection and autoimmune disorders.

The main potential risks might paradoxically centre on the exquisite ability of MSCs to suppress immune responses, which may promote a state of immune deficiency leading to infection or activation of benign tumours (Djouad et al., 2003). Another concern is whether administered MSCs promote the growth of a latent tumor. MSC can be recruited to the stroma of developing tumors when systemically infused in animal models for glioma, colon carcinoma, ovarian carcinoma, Karposi's sarcoma and melanoma. Other detrimental effects might involve the ability of MSCs to migrate to tumours, which could lead to reciprocal interactions between MSCs and malignant cells thus promoting tumour growth and metastasis (Karnoub et al.,2007). A further tumourigenic risk may be associated with extensive in vitro culture of MSCs, which has been shown to initiate cytogenetic abnormalities and subsequent tumour formation upon transplantation in murine hosts. However, there is increasing evidence that with respect to the risk of MSCs transformation and subsequent tumor formation initiated by MSCs, human MSCs appear to be safe. Therefore we feel impelled to strongly recommend at this point careful quality control procedures for all cell preparations. These should be implemented for all kinds of cell-based therapies. Suffice it to say that before administering MSCs to patients the cell preparations have to undergo careful phenotypic, functional, and genetic characterizations.

In conclusion, the record of safety for MSCs in general is excellent and we anticipate that after successful conclusion of ongoing preclinical and clinical tests, MSCs will be gradually introduced into clinical practice for a number of disease conditions in the coming years. Careful pre-administration safety monitoring as well as close monitoring of the patients are important pre-requisites for the success of this novel form of therapy. Regulatory bodies such as the US Food and Drug administration and the European Union have recently established a set of regulations for cell-based therapeutics. With continuous and open interactions between investigators, research institutions and regulatory bodies, successful, and most importantly, safe cell-based therapies will become routine for patients' treatment in the near future.

7. Acknowledgment

The authors gratefully acknowledge the expert technical assistance provided by Fan-Ming Kong, Xiao-Ping Xue, and Xiu-Zhu Yang

8. References

Al-Abdullah IH, Ayala T, Panigrahi D, Kumar RM, Kumar MS(2000). Neogenesis of pancreatic endocrine cells in copper-deprived rat models. *Pancreas;* 21: 63–68.

Barry FP, Murphy JM(2004). Mesenchymal stem cells: clinical applications and biological characterization. *Int J Biochem Cell Biol;* 36:568-84.

Bonner-Weir S, Taneja M, Weir GC, et al(2000). In vitro cultivation of human islets from expanded ductal tissue. *ProcNatlAcadSciUSA;*97:7999–8004.

Bonner-Weir S, Sharma A(2002). Pancreatic stem cells. *J Pathol;*197(4):519–26.

Bonner-Weir S, Baxter LA, Schuppin GT, Smith FE(1993). A second pathway for regeneration of adult exocrine and endocrine pancreas. A possible recapitulation of embryonic development. *Diabetes;* 42: 1715–1720.

Davidson PM, Campbell IL, Oxbrow L, Hutson JM, HarrisonLC(1989). Pancreatic beta cell proliferation in rabbits demonstrated by bromodeoxyuridine labeling. Pancreas,4:594–600.

Djouad, F., Plence, P., Bony, C., et al. (2003). Immunosuppressive effect of mesnechymal stem cells favors tumor growth in allogeneic animals. *Blood,* 102, 3837–3844.

Elsasser HP, Adler G, Kern HF(1986). Time course and cellular source of pancreatic regeneration following acute pancreatitis in the rat. *Pancreas;* 1: 421–429.

Fendrich V, Esni F, Garay MV, et al(2008). Hedgehog signaling is required for effective regeneration of exocrine pancreas. *Gastroenterology;*135:621–631.

Granger, A., and Kushner, J.A. (2009). Ductal Origin Hypothesis of Pancreatic Regeneration under Attack. *J. Intern. Med.* 266, 325–338.

Gu D, Sarvetnick N(1993). Epithelial cell proliferation and islet neogenesis in IFN-g transgenic mice. *Development;* 118:33–46.

Gu D, Lee MS, Krahl T, Sarvetnick N(1994). Transitional cells in the regenerating pancreas. *Development;* 120: 1873–1881.

Gu D, Arnush M, Sarvetnick N(1997). Endocrine/exocrine intermediate cells in streptozotocin-treated Ins-IFN- gamma transgenic mice. *Pancreas;* 15: 246–250.

Gu G, Brown JR, Melton DA(2003). Direct lineage tracing reveals the ontogeny of pancreatic cell fates during mouse embryogenesis. *Mech Dev;*120(1):35–43.

Gurda GT, Guo L, Lee SH, et al(2008). Cholecystokinin activates pancreatic calcineurin-NFAT signaling in vitro and in vivo. *Mol Biol Cell;*19:198–206.

Hanley NA, Hanley KP, Miettinen PJ, et al(2008). Weighing up beta-cell mass in mice and humans: selfrenewal, progenitors or stem cells? *Mol Cell Endocrinol;*288(12):79–85.

Holland A M., LJ G´o˜nez & Leonard C. Harrison(2004).Progenitor cells in the adult pancreas. *Diabetes Metab Res Rev;* 20: 13–27.

Horwitz EM, Prockop DJ, Gordon PL, Koo WWK, Fitzpatrick LA, Neel MD, McCarville ME, Orchard PJ, Pyeritz RE, Brenner MK(2001). Clinical responses to bone marrow transplantation in children with severe osteogenesis imperfecta. *Blood,* 97:1227-1231.

Karnoub, A. E., Dash, A. B., Vo, A. P., et al. (2007).Mesenchymal stem cells within tumour stroma promote breast cancer metastasis. *Nature,* 449, 557–563.

Kelly L, Reid L, Walker NI(1999). Massive acinar cell apoptosis with secondary necrosis, origin of ducts in atrophic lobules and failure to regenerate in cyanohydroxybutene pancreatopathy in rats. *Int J Exp Pathol;* 80: 217–226.

Koc ON, Day J, Nieder M, Gerson SL, Lazarus HM, Krivit W(2002). Allogeneic mesenchymal stem cell infusion for treatment of metachromatic leukodystrophy (MLD) and Hurler syndrome (MPS-IH). *Bone Marrow Transplantation;*30:215-222.

Kritzik MR, Jones E, Chen Z, *et al(*1999). PDX-1 and Msx-2 expression in the regenerating and developing pancreas. *J Endocrinol;* 163: 523–530.

Like AA, Rossini AA(1976). Streptozotocin-induced pancreatic insulitis: new model of diabetes mellitus. *Science;* 193:415–417.

Minami K, Okuno M, Miyawaki K, et al(2005). Lineage tracing and characterization of insulin-secreting cells generated from adult pancreatic acinar cells. *Proc Natl Acad Sci U S A,* 102(42):15116–21.

O'Reilly LA, Gu D, Sarvetnick N, *et al(*1997). Alpha-Cell neogenesis in an animal model of IDDM. *Diabetes;* 46: 599–606.

Pittenger, G.L., Taylor-Fishwick, D., and Vinik, A.I. (2009). A role for islet neogenesis in curing diabetes. *Diabetologia,* 52(5):735-8.

Prockop DJ, Olson SD(2007). Clinical trials with adult stem/progenitor cells for tissue repair: Let's not overlook some essential precautions. *Blood,*109:3147-3151.

Rafaeloff R, Pittenger GL, Barlow SW, *et al(* 1997). Cloning and sequencing of the pancreatic islet neogenesis associated protein (INGAP) gene and its expression in islet neogenesis in hamsters. *J Clin Invest;* 99: 2100–2109.

Sandgren EP, Luetteke NC, Palmiter RD, Brinster RL, Lee DC(1990). Overexpression of TGF alpha in transgenic mice: induction of epithelial hyperplasia, pancreatic metaplasia, and carcinoma of the breast. *Cell;* 61: 1121–1135.

Schofield R(1978). The relationship between the spleen colonyforming cell and the haemopoietic stem cell. *Blood Cells;*4: 7–25.

Sharma A, Zangen DH, Reitz P, *et al(* 1999). The homeodomain protein IDX-1 increases after an early burst of proliferation during pancreatic regeneration. *Diabetes;* 48: 507–513.

Siveke JT, Lubeseder-Martellato C, Lee M, et al(2008). Notch signaling is required for exocrine regeneration after acute pancreatitis. *Gastroenterology;*134:544–555.

Song SY, Gannon M,Washington MK, *et al(*1999*)*. Expansion of Pdx1-expressing pancreatic epithelium and islet neogenesis in transgenic mice overexpressing transforming growth factor alpha. *Gastroenterology;* 117: 1416–1426.

Trento C, Dazzi F *(*2010*)*. Mesenchymal stem cells and innate tolerance: biology and clinical applications. *Swiss Med Wkly.;*140:w13121

Waguri M, Yamamoto K, Miyagawa JI, *et al(1997)*. Demonstration of two different processes of beta-cell regeneration in a new diabetic mousemodel induced by selective perfusion of alloxan. *Diabetes;* 46: 1281–1290.

Wang RN, Kloppel G, Bouwens L*(*1995). Duct- to islet-cell differentiation and islet growth in the pancreas of duct-ligated adult rats. *Diabetologia;* 38: 1405–1411.

Wolfe-Coote S, Louw J, Woodroof C, Du Toit DF *(*1996). The non-human primate endocrine pancreas: development, regeneration potential and metaplasia. *Cell Biol Int;* 20:95–101.

Xia B, Zhan XR, Yi R, et al(2009). Can pancreatic duct-derived progenitors be a source of islet regeneration? *Biochem Biophys Res Commun;*383(4):383–385.

Yamaoka T, Yoshino K, Yamada T, *et al(* 2000). Diabetes and tumor formation in transgenic mice expressing reg I. *Biochem Biophys Res Commun;* 278: 368–376.

2

Gene Therapy Approach: HSV-Enkephalin Reduces Fibrosis, Inflammation, and Pain

Karin N. Westlund
University of Kentucky Medical Center, USA

1. Introduction

Chronic alcohol abuse is a major precipitating cause of pancreatitis along with genetic predisposition. Chronic alcohol and alcohol metabolite exposure can produce profound pancreatic tissue destruction in addition to damaging effects to other organs (Apte et al., 2009; Pezzilli et al., 2009). Pancreatitis causes over 2,000 deaths per year and over 100,000 hospitalizations. Acute initial attacks can be fatal and about 20% of these elevate to chronic conditions which are irreversible. Chronic pancreatitis places patients at 50-60% increased risk of progressing to pancreatic cancer. Severe unmitigated pain is synonymous with pancreatic inflammation and cancer caused by fibrotic blockage of the ductal system, premature trypsin activation, inflammation, perineural damage and nerve exposure.

Pancreatitis is characterized by severe histopathological changes, such as the presence of inflammatory mediators, acinar atrophy, fat necrosis, intraductal hemorrhage, periductal fibrosis and stromal proliferation (Schmidt et al., 1995). Elevated serum α-amylase, lipase, and CRP levels serve as biochemical markers of acute pancreatitis (Merkord et al., 1997; Sparmann et al., 1997). Acute pancreatitis ranges from mild edematous conditions that usually heal without intervention, to severe hemorrhagic necrotizing inflammation that is often fatal over a period of days as patients succumb to abdominal sepsis and multi-organ failure (Schmidt et al., 1992; Vardanyan and Rilo, 2010). The level of pain experienced by these patients is directly linked to decreased pancreatic functioning and increased length of stay during hospitalizations. In patient surveys, 32% of patients in chronic pancreatitis pain report being willing to try any new therapy for relief, and some may resort to suicide for this intractable pain state. Thus, the need to pursue novel pain relief strategies remains high for patients with chronic pancreatitis pain and those with pancreatic cancer who now have increasingly longer survival times.

2. Acute and chronic pancreatitis models: histological features

We have examined several *in vivo* and *in vitro* models of alcohol injury in combination with a gene therapy approach to examine ability to reduce the consequences of alcohol related injury. An acute inflammatory pancreatitis is induced in rats with a noxious chemical, dibutyltin dichloride, used in fertilizers and plastics manufacturing. A chronic pancreatitis is induced by maintenance on a high fat and alcohol (6%) diet. Both the chemical and the diet induced pancreatitis models produce histologically evident damage to the chymotrypsin producing acinar cells, inflammatory cell invasion and activation, interstitial edema, cell swelling and proliferation of local tissue stellate immune cells within the pancreas (**Fig. 1**; Lu et al., 2007; Yang et al., 2008).

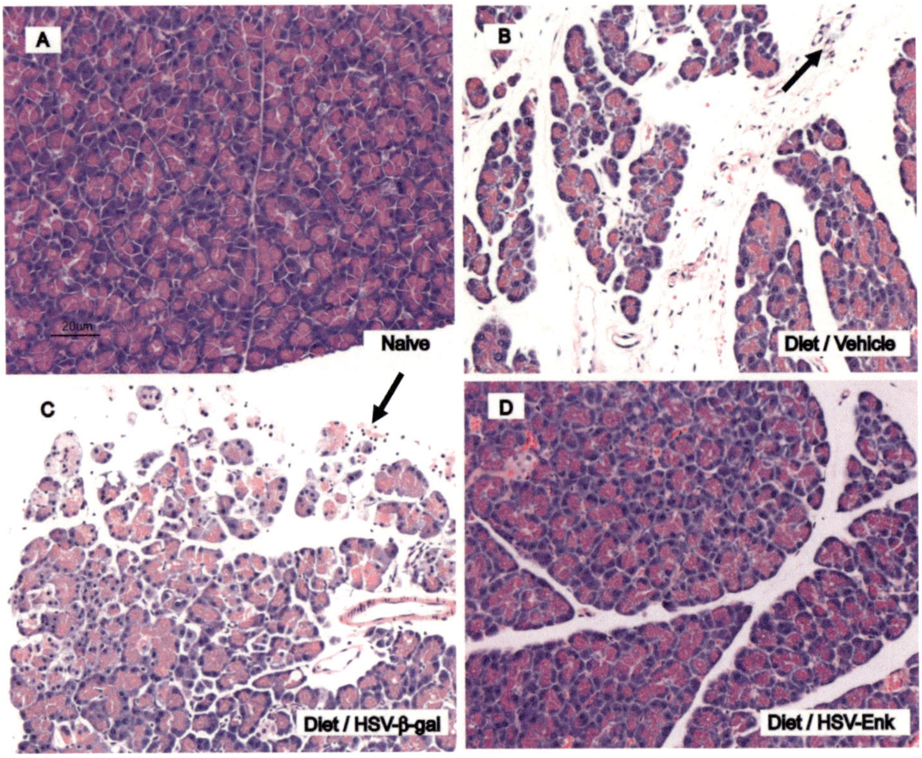

Fig. 1. **Histopathology of rat pancreas at week 10**. **A**. Naïve animals were fed low soy chow and given no treatment. **B**. Method control animals given the alcohol (6%) and high-fat diet to induce pancreatitis were given pancreatic injection of vehicle (DMEM) only. **C**. Some animals with alcohol and high-fat diet induced pancreatitis were given pancreatic HSV-β-gal applications, serving as the vector control. Note the steatosis, inflammatory cell infiltration (arrows), acinar cell necrosis, tissue edema, ductal widening and periductal fibrosis seen in the controls, with alcohol and high-fat diet induced pancreatitis given vehicle or the HSV-β-gal applications (**B** and **C**). **D**. Greatly reduced inflammatory cell infiltration and preservation of pancreatic tissue architecture was seen in animals fed the alcohol and high-fat diet but treated with the HSV-ENK vector. The histopathology of the HSV-ENK vector treated animals was similar to that of the naïve animals (**A**). Hemotoxylin and eosin (H&E) stain. (Reprinted from Yang et al., 2008)

3. Acute and chronic pancreatitis models: pain related behaviors

These pancreatitis models also produce pain related behaviors. The novel open field test box revealed significant reductions in active behavioral measures (exploratory rearing; beam breaks; active time, duration, distance traveled), as well as increased rest time for animals with acute pancreatitis (**Fig. 2**).

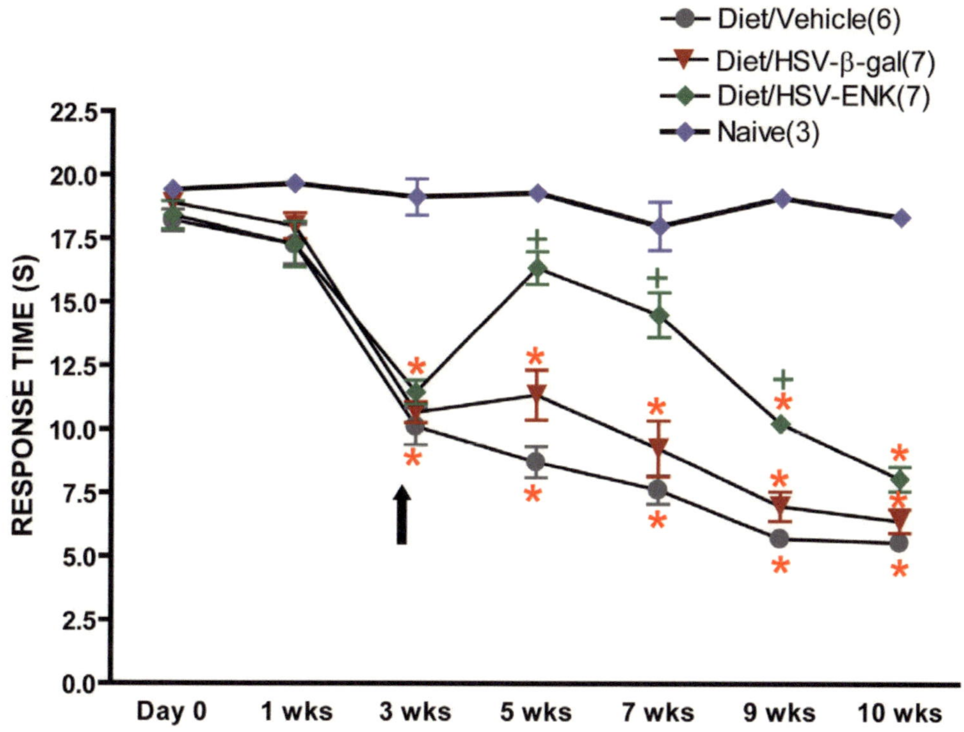

Hotplate test of thermal sensitivity for naive rats or rats with pancreatitis given either vehicle, HSV-ENK, or HSV-β-gal treatment. *$p \leq 0.05$, vs Day0 (Mann Whitney U test); +$p \leq 0.05$, Diet/HSV-Enk group vs Diet/Vehicle (Mann Whitney U test).

Fig. 2. **Hot plate response latency nociceptive behavior measurements.** Hot plate response latency measurements are shown for naïve animals and animal groups with alcohol and high-fat induced pancreatitis. Hot plate test was conducted at baseline before induction of pancreatitis and for ten weeks subsequently. Note the significant shortening of hot plate response latencies for rats on the high fat and alcohol diet after week 3, indicating sensitization. The HSV-ENK treatment (arrow) significantly abrogated the shift in response latency for at least four weeks. Four weeks is typical of HSV vector expression. (Reprinted from Yang et al., 2008)

4. Opiate gene therapy studies

In initial fMRI studies using the acute DBTC induced pancreatitis model, we determined levels of neuronal activation in higher brain centers along the visceral pain pathway (Westlund, 2000) finding significant activation in rostral ventrolateral medulla, dorsal raphe, periaqueductal grey, medial thalamus and central amygdala in rats (Westlund et al., 2009).

The pancreatitis induced brain activation was reduced by administration of morphine. Thus, we subsequently studied reduction of histological and behavioral consequences of the Herpes viral vectors (HSV-1) that overexpress the precursor of the endogenous opiate met-enkephalin in both the acute and chronic pancreatitis models. The gene therapy approach was used to overexpress the precursor for the endogenous opiate peptide met-enkephalin and was found to provide histological and behavioral mitigation of the histological **(Fig. 1D)** and behavioral changes (**Fig. 2**) induced by the pancreatitis. Met-enkephalin is an opioid growth factor known to increase wound healing and restore homeostasis in the cornea (Sassani et al., 2003).

The chronic high fat diet and alcohol-induced pancreatitis allowed study of the full time course for enkephalin's effectiveness (6 weeks) after a single inoculation directly into the pancreas (Yang et al., 2008; Westlund, 2009a). Met-enkephalin gene therapy is effective in the chronic alcohol diet induced pancreatitis model, as well as in an acute chemically induced model for reduction of tissue injury, fibrosis, inflammation, and pain-related behaviors (Lu et al., 2007; Yang et al., 2008; Westlund, 2009a). The fibrosis was abundant in animals with chronic pancreatitis and was stainable with picrosirius (overnight 0.1% Sirius red) as an addition to hemotoxylin/eosin histology (**Fig. 3,** right). Fibrosis produced by activated stellate cells characterizes the model as a chronic condition since it can lead to ductal stenosis that is one of the primary causes of pain for patients with pancreatitis. Histological data demonstrates that the proenkephalin gene product delivery to pancreas is reparative (**Fig. 1D**).

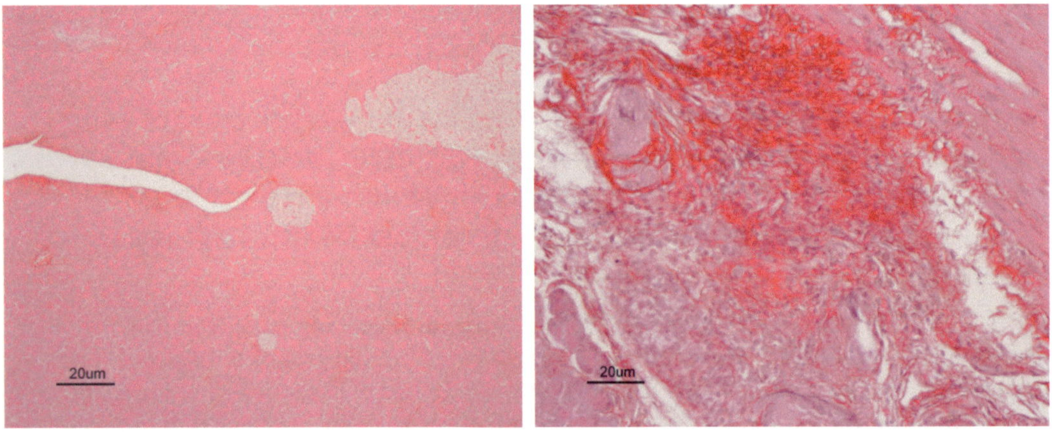

Fig. 3. **Alcohol and high fat diet induced pancreatic fibrosis.** Histological features evident in control pancreatic tissues (left) were severely disrupted in animals with chronic pancreatitis fed the high fat and alcohol diet (right). Fibrosis evident with Sirius red staining was abundant in the animals with pancreatitis and was less dense in animals given the HSV-1 proenkephalin viral vector.

Staining for met-enkephalin is elevated only in the group treated with the HSV-ENK overexpression vector in chronic alcohol diet fed rats after 10 weeks (**Fig. 4, 5**), as well as in the chemically induced pancreatitis at one week. Immunohistochemical localization of the HSV-1 proenkephalin overexpression product, met-enkephalin, was identified in abundance in both the spinal cord (**Fig. 4D**) and the pancreas (**Fig. 5D**). Levels of met-enkephalin in

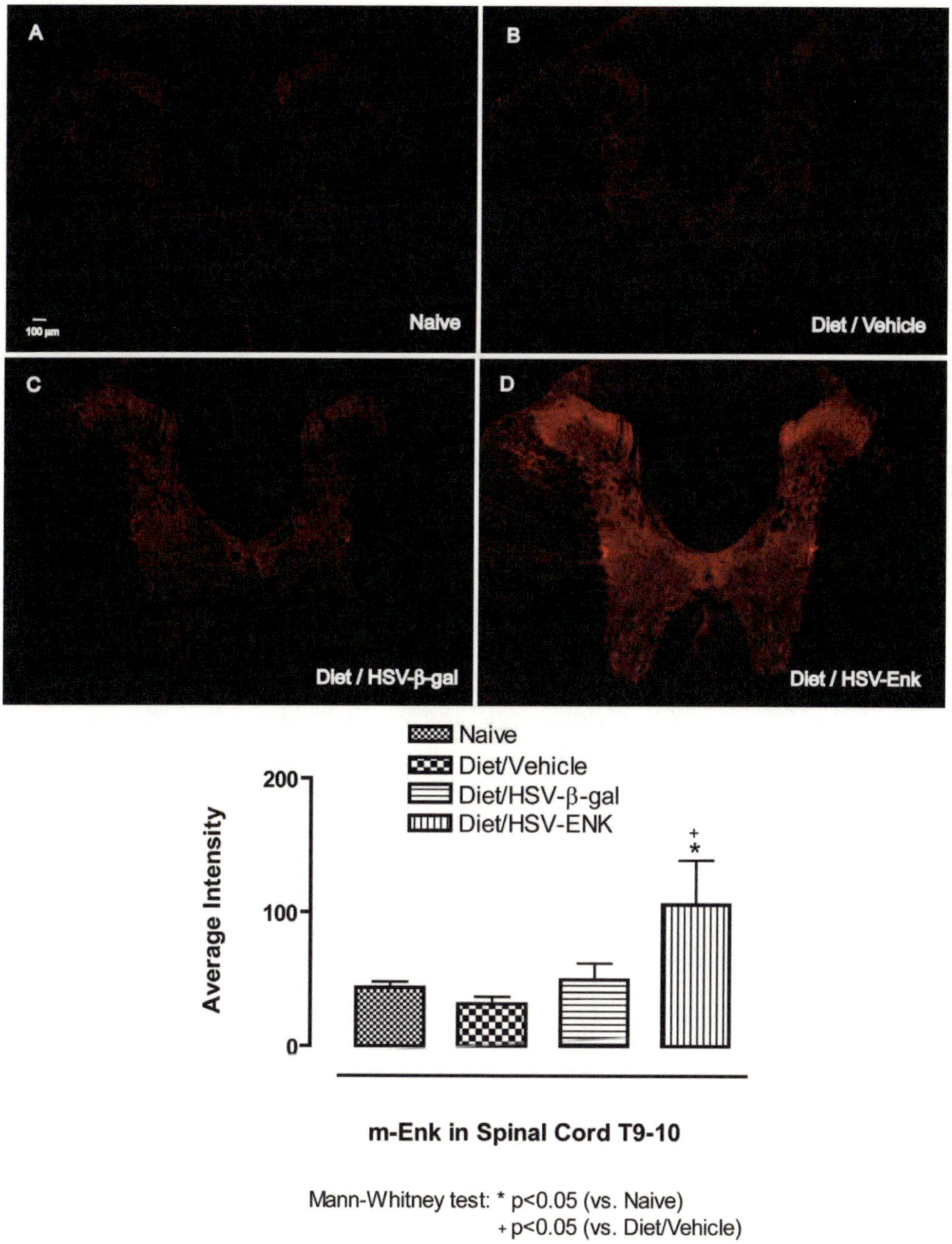

Fig. 4. **met-Enkephalin immunohistochemical staining in spinal cord (T9–10).** **A.** The spinal cord from a naïve rat is shown for comparison to (**B**) the spinal cord of animals with diet-induced pancreatitis at week 10. **C.** The expression of met-ENK after application of vehicle or HSV-β-gal is similar to naïve rats (**A**). **D.** Met-ENK expression was significantly increased in HSV-ENK vector-treated animals compared to controls. Met-ENK in the dorsal horn (laminae I–II) of the thoracic spinal cord was increased bilaterally. (Reprinted from Yang et al., 2008)

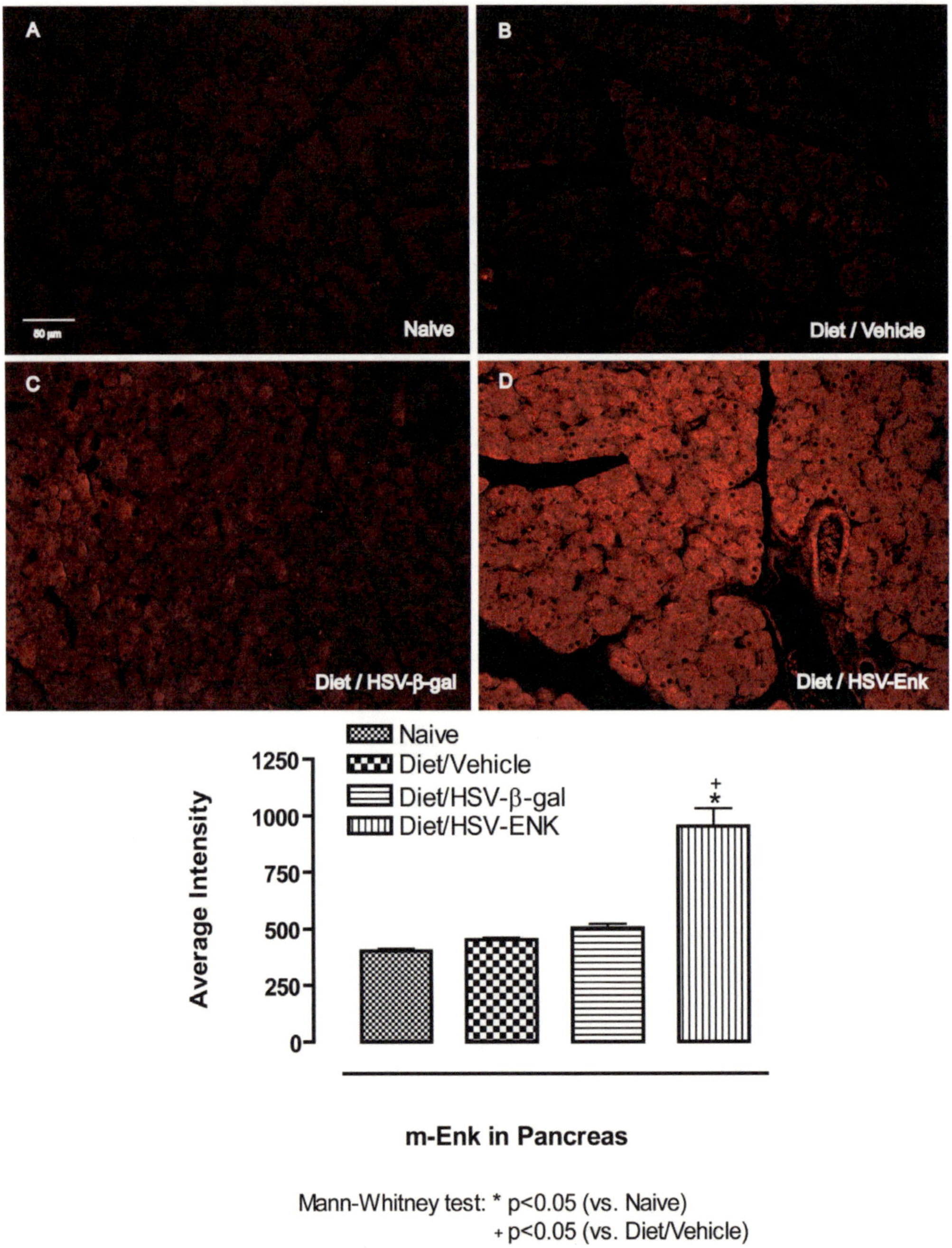

Fig. 5. **met-Enkephalin immunohistochemical staining in pancreas**. Photomicrographs and quantification of immunohistochemical staining for met-enkephalin in pancreas are shown for week 10. Minimal or no staining is seen in pancreas of (**A**) naïve and (**B-C**) control animals with alcohol and high-fat diet induced pancreatitis. **D**. Met-ENK expression was significantly increased in the pancreas of HSV-ENK-treated animals fed the same diet compared to the controls. (Reprinted from Yang et al., 2008)

pancreas were measured in a small number of animals with HPLC after one week of acute DBTC-induced pancreatitis. Levels, barely detectable in control pancreas, increase to about 3500ng/ml after one week of met-enkephalin overexpression. No staining for met-enkephalin was evident in naïve, vehicle or in animals receiving control viral vector (**Fig. 4A-C, 5A-C**).

There is negligible RANTES staining in naïve controls (**Fig 6A**) or animals with pancreatitis after met-enkephalin overexpression (**Fig 6D**) with either model indicating met-enkephalin protects the pancreas from effects of invading inflammatory cells. Staining for the inflammatory mediator RANTES is clearly evident in the pancreas in vehicle- and HSV-β-gal-treated animals with pancreatitis at week 10 (**Fig 6B and 6C**, respectively) at week 10. Both acinar cells and infiltrating inflammatory cells were positive for RANTES and COX-2 at one week (not shown).

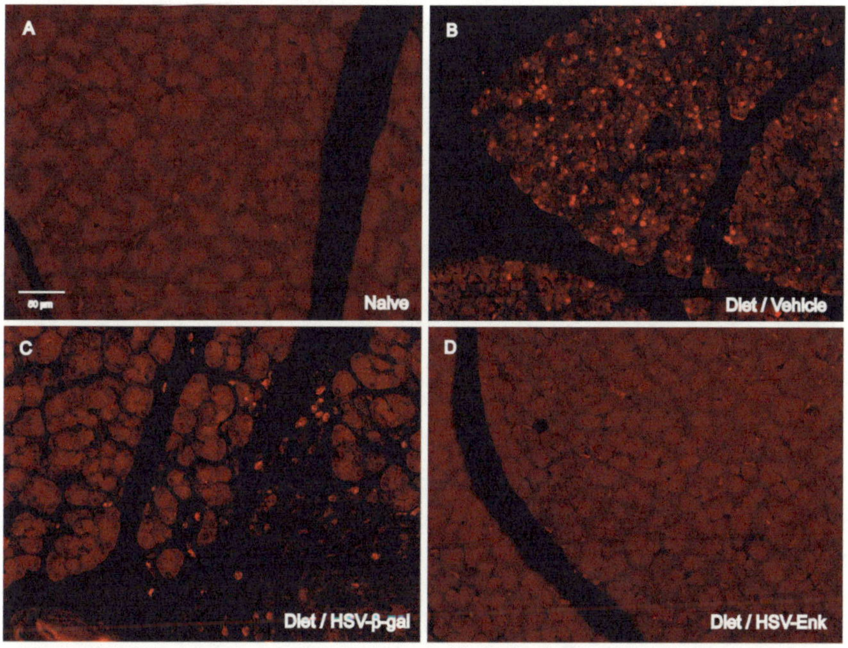

Fig. 6. **RANTES immunohistochemical staining in pancreas.** Photomicrographs of immunohistochemical staining of RANTES in the pancreas of rats are shown for week 10. A. Naïve rat pancreas. B. Diet-induced pancreatitis and application of vehicle as control. C. Diet-induced pancreatitis and application of the HSV-β-gal control vector. D. Animals given the same diet and application of HSV-ENK. Note the increased RANTES staining in pancreata of animals with alcohol and high-fat diet induced pancreatitis treated with vehicle or HSV-β-gal applications. Little or no staining of RANTES is noted in naïve and HSV-ENK-treated animals. (Reprinted from Yang et al., 2008)

We propose that met-enkephalin is acting as a protective/restorative agent against pancreatic insult. Met-enkephalin acts on μ-opioid receptors that we observed in pancreatic acinar and stellate cells in our chemically induced pancreatitis model (Lu et al., 2007). Increased expression of μ-opioid receptors was detected in the pancreas with the DBTC induced acute pancreatitis at one week. The μ-opioid receptors induced in pancreas by DBTC pancreatitis are reduced by HSV-enkephalin except in stellate cells (Lu et al., 2007).

In our studies, HSV-ENK injected rats with pancreatitis have normal or nearly normal responses to noxious heat (**Fig. 2**). Opioid peptides generated from three precursor genes, proenkephalin, prodynorphin and POMC, are conserved phylogenetically (Salzet, 2001). The mechanism of action for reduction of pain related behaviors in this and previous studies are likely related to enkephalin's influence directly both on the central and the peripheral opioid receptors by the overexpressed met-enkephalin at those sites (**Figures 4, 5**). Proenkephalin derived opioid peptides are released peripherally after HSV-ENK administration (Yeomans et al., 2006). Their effect would mimic the enhanced endogenous release of opiates from immune cells that invade the region of inflammation and modulate both pain and inflammatory parameters (Stein, 1995). While many of the opiate peptides are delivered by inflammatory cells drawn to sites of inflammation, opioid neuropeptides may be more prominent in influencing nociceptive signaling when delivered at the synaptic endings. Proenkephalin gene product met-enkephalin is expressed in a 3:1 ratio relative to proenkephalin gene product, leu-enkephalin. The factors regulating why some gene products from the opioid families have more efficient translational processing, or are expressed in greater ratios is not completely understood (Danielson and Dores, 1999). The proenkephalin viral construct is chosen for proposed gene therapy pain studies since it is more prominent in influencing nociception.

The opioid-mediated anti-hyperalgesia of HSV-ENK infected animals mimics the effects of endogenous or intrathecally administered enkephalin in our hands. However, enkephalins are very labile and the natural neuronal ending release provided by the HSV-1 viral vector is a superior release method. In a cutaneous inflammation model, HSV-ENK infected animals were no different from controls suggesting that opioids are not tonically released, but are released only when there is a substantial activation of the afferents providing evidence that hyperalgesia can be blocked without altering baseline nociception (Wilson et al., 1999).

Our studies were equally successful with replication conditional or replication defective viral constructs. Both effectively reduce nociceptive behaviors in our models and in somatic pain models in previous studies (Wilson et al., 1999) but have no effect in control animals. Previous studies of HSV-1 transgene therapy have been used successfully to assess the anti-nociceptive effects of transduced opioids in inflammatory models, including experimental models of cutaneous inflammation and polyarthritis (Braz et al., 2001; Wilson et al., 1999; Wilson and Yeomans, 2000; Wilson and Yeomans, 2002). In the previous studies, application of HSV-1 virus vector containing a human proenkephalin gene resulted in transmission by viral spread through primary afferent fibers into the dorsal root ganglia. Subsequent protein expression from the proenkephalin or ß-galactosidase gene (control neutral protein) could be visualized in the spinal cord (Wilson et al., 1999). Human proenkephalin-encoding HSV-1 viral vector reduced hyperalgesia by 60% in a polyarthritis model (Braz et al., 2001). Histological and behavioral effects were observed at 4-9 days post-infection (Wilson et al, 1999). The maximal response after hindpaw application of HSV-1 enkephalin-coding viral vector was reported at 14 days (Braz et al., 2001). Both of these studies validate that time is required for incorporation of viral vectors into nerve terminals, for retrograde transport of the viral vector to the DRG, and for subsequent peptide production.

Additional findings in the experimental polyarthritis model reported by Braz and colleagues (2001) was clear radiographic evidence that the animals receiving the HSV enkephalin gene encoding viral vectors also sustained significantly less joint destruction than the control animals after CFA injection. Both studies demonstrated that the opioid receptor antagonist, naloxone, delivered subcutaneously or intrathecally, could partially or completely restore sensitization in the HSV-1 enkephalin encoding vector infected animals but had no effect on HSV-1-ß-galactosidase encoding vector or mock infected animals. This suggests opioid mediation of observed anti-nociceptive effects and suggests that the effect was in part due to spinal release of opioids. Naloxone methiodide administration increased hyperalgesia in animals infected with HSV-ENK when administered for three days (Braz et al., 2001). In another model, HSV-ENK delivery by intradermal application was as effective in controlling pain related measures as intrathecal administration of enkephalin (Wilson et al., 1999). These and our studies are compelling in that HSV-1 opioid gene delivery potentially offers a significantly sustained response (up to 7 weeks) in the experimental rodent models. **Thus, analgesia and restorative effects of HSV-Enk gene therapy will likely be effective in both somatic and visceral clinical pain.**

5. Viral vectors: analgesic and anti-inflammatory potential

Few studies to date report effective decreases in ongoing visceral pain with pharmacological treatments other than with opiates. Activation of opiate receptors leads to potent analgesia (Schafer et al., 1998), and opiates remain the primary therapeutic agent despite significant side effects and development of tolerance. Gene therapy is a novel drug delivery system capable of bringing over-expressed opiates directly to pancreatic tissues. The site specific delivery of HSV-1 viral vectors, which have an affinity for uptake by primary sensory neuronal endings (neurotropic), provided the preferable gene delivery construct for visceral anti-nociception. Wild type HSV-1 is a 154 Kb neurotropic double stranded DNA virus, containing 84 essential and nonessential viral genes. After natural primary cutaneous or mucosal inoculation, viral particles enter sensory axon terminals innervating the affected area. They are carried by retrograde axonal transport from the periphery to DRG, where the virus may establish a life-long latent state (Burton et al., 2001; Steiner et al., 1990). For gene therapy applications, the modified HSV-1 nucleocapsid and tegument can also use the same transport mechanism for successful passage to DRG. Modified viruses have been constructed and used successfully in many pre-clinical studies and Phase I/II clinical trials. Results of trials are published at www.oxtl.com. In one strategy, replication defective viral constructs have deletions of essential immediate early genes from the HSV-1 genome. In another strategy, replication conditional viruses are generated by insertion of the desired gene into the HSV-1 genes required for productive infections (i.e. thymidine kinase gene).

A recent Phase I clinical trial administered a replication defective HSV vector similar to the one given in our studies to upregulate proenkephalin (Wolfe et al., 2009b). The clinical report indicates that the vector provided significant pain relief for 12–24 patients with intractable focal pain from terminal cancer.

There are several inherent advantages to using HSV based viral constructs for foreign gene delivery in certain clinical settings, rather than other viral delivery models under study. The inserted genes are under the control of a strong constitutive human cytomegalovirus promoter (hCMV), which **allows expression of inserted gene product at an intracellular locale, in the absence of productive HSV-1 infection and without integration into the host genome** (Wilson et al., 1999). The recombinant viral vectors designed for gene therapy rendered replication conditional or defective do not produce productive viral infection *in vivo,* but can persist for months despite negligible viral protein synthesis. These viral constructs establish a quiescent state similar to natural viral latency but **cannot reactivate to cause active infection in neuronal cells** *in vivo* (Goins et al., 2001; Wilson et al., 1999; Wilson and Yeomans, 2002). Lentiviruses as vectors offer very efficient infection, gene expression in activated cells and genome integration into host DNA for gene replacement therapy. However, current lentiviral constructs result in systemic infection and cannot be contained and the site of lentiviral insertion into the host genome cannot be controlled.They are considered a potential causal agent of cancers, autoimmune diseases and acquired immune deficiency syndrome (AIDS). Potential concerns exist regarding development of helper phenonoma for unwanted expressions and genetic recombination with other lentiviruses, including those already integrated in the host genome. Viral construct design for adenoviruses has also yielded promising results, but adenoviruses may not be advantageous since they can also involve the central nervous system.

HSV-1 viral constructs may offer unique advantages in peripheral inflammation, as they selectively infect primary sensory neurons but do not integrate into the host genome. Thus, they will be an independent "minipump" source for protein synthesis in the neuronal cytoplasm. As a DNA-based viral construct, (1) the rate of mutation and recombination in these HSV-1 constructs will be minimal to nonexistent since (2) these constructs do not enter into productive infection or latency phases. Further, preliminary data suggest that HSV replication deficient viral constructs do not generate proteins that would induce an amnestic response from the host, activating latent prior HSV-1 infection. These are very important properties of HSV-1 based viral vectors, as 70-90% of the human adult population has evidence of prior HSV-1 infection. This limited potential to generate a host response also improves the potential for using repeated dosings of HSV-based viral constructs. Adenoviruses cause productive infection, induce host inflammation above the inflammation already generated in target tissues and increase potential for extended injury and host innate immune response to the virus making repeated doses problematic (Minter et al., 2001).

Local injection of HSV-1 viral construct with human proenkephalin gene insert results in targeted tissue expression of opioid protein (Yeomans et al., 2006), whereas systemic administration of some neural agents have undesirable or intolerable side effects (Goss et al., 2002). HSV-1 gene delivery and local opioid expression may potentiate exogenously administered morphine, lowering doses needed and delaying morphine tolerance (Stein et al., 1996). This has been demonstrated in other HSV-based gene therapy models, where HSV-viral vector infections potentiated chemotherapy agents in lung cancer (Toyoizumi et al., 1999) and breast cancer (Thomas and Fraser, 2003). Attenuated herpes simplex viruses have already been successfully used in Phase I/II trials for treatment of CNS glioblastoma without apparent nonspecific toxic effects (Papanastassiou et al., 2002). The efficacy and potency of peripheral opioid effects are generally enhanced when drugs are administered during active inflammatory conditions (Antonijevic et al., 1995; Lamigeon et al., 2001; Schafer et al., 1998; Stein, 1995; Walker, 2003).

6. Anti-inflammatory effects and tissue protection by HSV-Enk treatment

It is well known that long term administration of morphine reduces immune function through reduced hypothalamic-pituitary-adrenal axis activation. Opioid receptors are constitutively expressed in non-neuronal sites including vascular endothelial cells (Cadet et al., 2000 and Saeed et al., 2000), on immune cells such as macrophages and lymphocytes (Gavériaux et al., 1995), and keratinocytes (Bigliardi et al., 2002). A role for neuronal opiates has also been shown for reduction of inflammation (for review see Machelska and Stein, 2003). While the role/s of specific extra-neuronal peripheral opioid receptors has not been fully established, mu (morphine), kappa (U50488H) and delta-2 (deltorphin II), but not delta-1 (DPDPE) opioid agonists have been shown to produce dose-dependent immunosuppressive effects on a plaque-forming assay, effects that were blocked by respective selective opioid antagonists (Rahim et al., 2001). It is also well established that the spinal cord can regulate peripheral inflammation through a variety of dorsal horn receptor mechanisms and retrograde primary afferent activity (Rees et al., 1994; Ren and Dubner, 1999; Sluka et al., 1993; Sluka et al., 1994; Sluka and Westlund, 1993; Sorkin et al., 2003). This includes glutamate, GABA, substance P and adenosine receptor mechanisms likely influenced by opiates (Boyle et al., 2002). Much less well studied is the report that mu opiates can directly reduce plasma extravasation ((24-36%) Joris et al., 1990; Binder et al., 2001; Green and Levine, 1992; Barber et al., 1993; Taylor et al., 2000). These effects are induced by activation of opioid receptors located in the central and peripheral nervous systems. In the periphery, opioid receptors are expressed on a significant proportion of capsaicin sensitive sensory fibers and sympathetic postganglionic terminals, where they may participate in the modulation of nociceptive information under certain pathological conditions (Zhou et al., 1998). The reversibility of the effects induced by the opioid receptor agonists (edema and extravasation) has been established after the administration of antagonists (i.p.) (Romero et al., 2005). The work of Lei and Rogers (1999) in intact respiratory tissue suggests that opioid receptors located on sensory fibers and immune cells are selectively activated by low (neuronal) or high (non-neuronal) doses of mu- and delta-opioid receptor agonists. The local administration of mu- and delta-opioid receptor agonists, at doses that show no systemic effect, has been shown to decrease plasma extravasation during peripheral inflammation (Hong and Abbott, 1995). This suggests a clinical application for low dose morphine or met-enk as a pre-emptive treatment to avoid endoscopic procedure induced pancreatitis. It is likely that a similar mechanism is reducing inflammatory signs in the HSV-ENK treated animals releasing enkephalin directly to the pancreas.

7. Development of opiate tolerance?

In our study, hyperalgesia in the control HSV-β-gal and vehicle treated animals with alcohol and high fat diet induced pancreatitis was maintained through seven weeks. The overexpression of the proenkephalin products in the HSV-ENK treated animals was sufficient to abrogate the effects of the pancreatitis for an extended period of time **without tolerance** demonstrating that this is an adequate model for treatment in clinical studies. The important issue of desensitization and tolerance to the enkephalin generated by the HSV-ENK construct, appears to be a non-issue in the time frame of study. We propose that it is the release of met-enkephalin directly onto receptors at nerve terminals both centrally and peripherally that provides additive effectiveness for reducing hyperalgesia and tissue protection from inflammatory responses without tolerance. In this site directed manner, enkephalin can affect receptors on neuronal endings that receive information about noxious conditions in the pancreas and have reparative ability as an apparent added benefit. Standard therapies relying on higher and higher levels of circulating opiates, on the other hand, frequently result in intolerable side-effects and development of tolerance. Gene therapy using HSV vectors for gene product delivery may be clinically preferred in patients with prospects of longer life spans and functionality, or in intractable chronic nonmalignant pancreatitis and generally indicated in patients with longer life spans. **HSV-1-based viral vector infections may offer a novel, effective, well-tolerated and advantageous approach for treatment of chronic pancreatic pain in patients. This approach might also be expanded to deliver additional human gene products that could impact the pain, inflammation, structural integrity and repair of the pancreas in patients.**

8. Testing safety and efficacy issues

Safety and efficacy of replication defective HSV vectors have already been demonstrated for other purposes in Phase 1 clinical trials (Todo, 2002; Shah 2003; Yu et al, 2004; Satoh, 2005; Sawai et al., 2001; Wolfe et al., 2009, a,b). For our studies we examined the spinal cord for evidence of HSV-1 infection after 12 weeks of study. While we expected and have demonstrated HSV-1 in the dorsal root ganglia sensory neurons (Yang et al., 2008), the preferred host cell for HSV, no central nervous system infection was found. This has not been tested in spinal cord previously with these viral vectors. The replication deficient virus has already been used safely when injected directly into the brain as a treatment for glioblastoma (Papanastassiou, et al., 2002). The efficacy and clinical relevance of the direct injection into the pancreas was successfully tested in our pre-clinical studies by examining behavioral, inflammatory and cellular activation responses, such as FOS protein expression in spinal neurons and phospho-p38 in DRG. Effects of met-enkephalin have also been tested in *in vitro* pancreatic cell models. We have infected DRG and pancreas cells in cultures (PANC-1) with HSV vectors to assess the longevity of enkephalin, inflammatory mediator release, re-activation and other safety issues in PANC-1 cells, clonal human pancreatic tumor-derived tubular epithelia equivalent to the cells lining the pancreatic ducts. The PANC-1 cells have been used previously by Eisenberg et al. (2005) to assess increased efficacy of HSV vectors used as an anti-cancer adjuvant to chemotherapeutic agents. In our studies the proenkephalin overexpression significantly reduced cytokine expression (unpublished data).

The phase I clinical trial using a related replication defective viral vector reported successful reduction of pain levels assessed using a numeric rating scale (NRS), the Short Form McGill Pain Questionnaire (SF-MPQ) and concurrent reduction of opiate usage in the terminal cancer patients initially with intractable pain (Wolfe et al., 2009b). The gene therapy studies provide compelling new insights in support of the effectiveness of enkephalin for reduction of tissue injury, fibrosis, inflammation, and pain related behaviors. The HSV viral system offers great potential for simultaneous delivery of multiple other gene products, as the HSV vector cassette is very large. Further improvement of vector system design may provide other anti-inflammatory gene products to protect and restore functional integrity of damaged tissues.

9. Clinical significance

As pancreatitis patient survival is becoming a fortunate reality, consideration of route of administration for viral constructs should be a part of investigative pre-clinical studies. While celiac plexus neurolysis is a currently accepted clinical treatment for severe intractable abdominal pain in abdominal malignancies and chronic pancreatitis, it is usually reserved for patients who have failed other treatment modalities. The reported year 1 success rate for pain relief is reportedly between 57-100%, depending on the approach and ethanol concentration (Okuyama et al., 2002; Vranken et al, 2002; Schmulewitz and Hawes, 2003; Klapman and Chang, 2005). Celiac plexus neurolysis requires surgical or anesthetic specialization and is usually performed at tertiary referral centers. Some procedural approaches require an epidural block for anesthesia. Although generally well-tolerated, reported complications include back pain, hypotension, and diarrhea (Chan, 1996; Kulke, 2002). Celiac plexus neurolysis essentially scleroses the nerve and blocks the afferent and efferent transmission of all neurochemicals. Neural blockade of a significant part of the enteric sympathetic nervous system in an otherwise functioning enteric system may lead to pancreatic or enteric pathologies, as the sympathetic nervous system plays a vital role in modulating intestinal secretory and absorptive processes. This may become more of an issue with the improved cancer treatments and longer lifespan for pancreatic malignancies. Viral vectors could be administered to coeliac ganglia in patients by anesthesiologists. However, it is not entirely clear that HSV-Enk would have sufficient uptake efficiency from the axons themselves as the primary afferents pass through the sympathetic ganglia and do not terminate there. We will compare sympathetic ganglia injections to administration at the pancreatic terminal endings which already appears to be quite robust. Our studies imply that chronic infusions of HSV vectors directly onto the pancreas surface from implantable, transcutaneously refillable pumps would provide relief from chronic pain. This potential treatment would also be nerve plexus sparing and avoid the severe complications of pancreatic duct disruption encountered by endoscopists. The sparing of neural connections would decrease the potential for pancreatic insufficiency and enteric damage.

Pancreatic cancer and chronic pancreatitis are among those syndromes characterized as causing the most severe pain states. Pancreatic cancer is the 4th leading cause of cancer deaths in the US, and over 70% of pancreatic cancer patients have significant debilitating abdominal pain upon clinical presentation. Over 50% of patients with idiopathic and alcoholic pancreatitis report chronic pain. The current treatment of pain in pancreatic cancer and chronic pancreatitis includes parenteral narcotic agents, surgical intervention at the level of pancreas or neural pathways and complementary therapies. Narcotic agents are not optimal as there are risks of tolerance, addiction and intolerable side effects of sedation and constipation and nausea. Surgical intervention with total pancreatectomy and islet autotransplantation provides pain relief for a considerable number of patients (Blondet et al., 2007; Hildebrand et al., 2011). However, surgery is invasive and can result in transient or suboptimal relief of pain, postoperative diabetes, and maldigestion. Surgery may be therapeutically or fiscally inappropriate based on the clinical status of some patients. Chronic abdominal pain from the pancreas has a significant negative long term impact on patient quality of life and mortality as it profoundly decreases appetite and leads to weight loss. When patients lose $\geq$20% of lean body mass, host immunocompetence is profoundly impaired. **Therefore, effective management of pain is imperative, not just for the legitimate concern for pain's sake, but for improvement in physical functioning, general health, patient survival, quality of life, and functional independence. Effective management of chronic pain would lift the economic burden of pain-induced debilitation on the individual, their support system and public health.**

Pain is a serious public health problem, costing the US about 100 billion dollars/yr (JAHCO report). Pain is the single greatest cause of disability, decreased physical function, decreased work productivity, absenteeism, reactive depression and lower quality of life (QOL, i.e. SF36) scores. In fact, 40-60% of patients with chronic pain report it has significantly and negatively impacted their personal relationships, work productivity and daily routines of living. Considerable improvements have been made in opioid medications, in term of bioavailability, half-life, transdermal delivery, breakthrough opioid combinations and usage with enhancing drugs, such as tricyclic antidepressants. However, side effects and potential for opioid addiction remain a concern to the patient, health care providers and the community. About 60% of patients with chronic pain have expressed fears regarding narcotic medication side effects and fear of addiction to current narcotic regimens. In a Partners Against Pain Survey of 1000 patients in chronic pain, 50% of the patients reported difficulty >1 yr in getting their pain under control and 78% of the patients reported that they would be willing to try new treatments.

Innovative Aspects of the Gene Therapy Studies

Unique advantages offered by HSV-1 viral vector delivery of proenkephalin expression products by the peripheral nerves include:

- Potential for simultaneous delivery of analgesic peptides to both peripheral and central sites, neuronal ending sites, optimizing the effects without tolerance
- More effective and prolonged abrogation of nociceptive responses
- Normalization of pain related behavior to near baseline levels as shown in the published studies
- Potential for positive impact on pancreatic inflammation as shown in the published studies
- HSV-1 viral constructs to be used are replication deficient/ defective
- HSV-1 viral constructs will not incorporate into the host genome or become lytic
- Focused delivery to the target organ allows a much lower viral titer (5-10X lower viral titer than in skin)
- Potential for reduction/elimination of the use of narcotic drugs
- Novel palliative strategy for alleviating the unremitting pain of pancreatic cancer and chronic pancreatitis

10. Conclusion

In summary, our studies indicate that the proenkephalin gene product delivery to pancreas is reparative and significantly reduce pain related behaviors in rodent pancreatitis models. Gene therapeutic approaches that promote the endogenous opiate enkephalin, particularly delivery by the neuronal innervation, may have significant clinical relevance for reducing inflammation, pain-related behavior and tissue destruction.

11. Acknowledgment

These studies were funded by NIH R01 NS039041. Acknowledgement is extended to Drs. Ying Lu and Hong Yang for their original study that is reviewed here through open access, as well as Drs. Sabrina McIlwrath and Liping Zhang for final edits.

12. References

Antonijevi, I.; Mousa, S.A.; Schafer, M. & Stein, C. (1995) Perineurial defect and peripheral opioid analgesia in inflammation. *Journal of Neuroscience*, Vol.15, pp.165-172.

Apte, M.; Pirola, R. & Wilson, J. (2009) New insights into alcoholic pancreatitis and pancreatic cancer. *Journal of Gastroenterology and Hepatology*. Vol.24, Suppl. 3, pp.S51-6.

Barber, A. (1993) μ and κ-opioid receptor agonists produce peripheral inhibition of neurogenic plasma extravasation in rat skin. *European Journal of Pharmacology*, Vol.236, pp.113–120.

Bigliardi, P.L.; Buchner, S.; Rufli, T. & Bigliardi-Qi, M. (2002) Specific stimulation of migration of human keratinocytes by mu-opiate receptor agonists. *Journal of Receptor Signaling and Transduction Research*, Vol.22, pp.191–199.

Binder, W.; Machelska, H.; Mousa, S.; Schmitt T, Rivière PJM, Junien JL, Stein C, Schäfer M (2001) Analgesic and antiinflammatory effects of two novel κ-opioid peptides. *Anesthesiology*, Vol. 94, pp.1034–1044.

Blondet, J.; Carlson, A.; Kobayashi, T.; Jie, T.; Bellin, M.; Hering, B.J.; Freeman, M.L.; Beilman, G.J. & Sutherland, D.E. (2007) The role of total pancreatectomy and islet autotransplantation for chronic pancreatitis. *Surgical Clinics of North America*, Vol.87, pp.1477-1501.

Boyle, D.L., Moore, J., Yang , L., Sorkin, L.S., Firestein, G.S. (2002) Spinal adenosine receptor activation inhibits inflammation and joint destruction in rat adjuvant-induced arthritis. *Arthritis and Rheumatology, Vol.* 46, pp.3076-3082.

Braz, J,; Beaufour, C.; Coutaux, A.; Epstein, A.L.; Cesselin, F.; Hamon, M. & Pohl, M. (2001) Therapeutic efficacy in experimental polyarthritis of viral-driven enkephalin overproduction in sensory neurons. *Journal of Neuroscience* 21: 7881-7888.

Burton, E.A.; Wechuck, J.B.; Wendell, S.K.; Goins, W.F.; Fink, D.J. & Glorioso, J.C. (2001) Multiple applications for replication-defective herpes simplex virus vectors. *Stem Cells* 19: 358-377.

Cadet P, Bilfinger, T.V.; Fimiani, C,; Peter, D. & Stefano, G.B. (2000) Human vascular and cardiac endothelia express mu opiate receptor transcripts. *Endothelium,* Vol.7, pp.185–191.

Chan, V.W. (1996) Chronic diarrhea: an uncommon side effect of celiac plexus block. *Anesthesia and Analgesia*. Ol. 82:205-7.

Danielson, P.B. & Dores, R.M. (1999) Molecular evolution of the opioid/orphanin gene family. *General Comparative Endocrinology*, Vol.113, pp. 169-186.

Eisenberg, D.P.; Adusumilli, P.S.; Hendershott, K.J.; Yu, Z.; Mullerad, M.; Chan, M.K.; Chou, T.C.; & Fong, Y. (2005) 5-fluorouracil and gemcitabine potentiate the efficacy of oncolytic herpes viral gene therapy in the treatment of pancreatic cancer. *Journal of Gastrointestinal Surgery*, Vol.9, pp.1068-77.

Gavériaux, C.; Peluso, J.; Simonin, F.; Laforet, J. & Kieffer, B. (1995) Identification of kappa- and delta-opioid receptor transcripts in immune cells. *FEBS Letters* Vol.369, pp.272–276.

Goins, W.F.; Yoshimura, N.; Phelan, M.W.; Yokoyama, T.; Fraser, M.O.; Ozawa, H.; Bennett, N., Jr.; de Groat, W.C.; Glorioso, J.C. & Chancellor, M.B. (2001) Herpes simplex virus mediated nerve growth factor expression in bladder and afferent neurons: potential treatment for diabetic bladder dysfunction. *Journal of Urology*, Vol.165, pp.1748-1754.

Goss, J.R.; Goins, W.F.; Lacomis, D.; Mata, M.; Glorioso, J.C. & Fink, D.J. (2002) Herpes simplex-mediated gene transfer of nerve growth factor protects against peripheral neuropathy in streptozotocin-induced diabetes in the mouse. *Diabetes*. Vol.51, No.7, pp.2227-3.

Green, P.G. & Levine, J.D. (1992) δ- and κ-opioid receptor agonists inhibit plasma extravasation induced by bradykinin in the knee joint of the rat. *Neuroscience*, Vol.49, pp.129–133.

Hildebrand, P.; Duderstadt, S.; Jungbluth, T.; Roblick, U.J.; Bruch, H.P. & Czymek, R. (2011) Evaluation of the quality of life after surgical treatment of chronic pancreatitis. *Journal of the Pancreas*, Vol.12, No.4, pp.364-71.

Hong, Y. & Abbott, F.V. (1995) Peripheral opioid modulation of pain and inflammation in the formalin test. *European Journal of Pharmacology*, Vol.277, pp.21–28.

Joris, J.; Costello, A., Dubner, R., Hargreaves, KkM (1990) Opiates suppress carrageenan-induced oedema and hyperthermia at doses that inhibit hyperalgesia. *Pain, Vol.*43, pp.95–103.

Klapman, J.B. & Chang, K.J. (2005) Endoscopic ultrasound-guided fine-needle injection. *Gastrointestinal Endoscopy Clinics North America*,Vol.15, pp.169-77.

Kulke, M.H. (2002) Metastatic pancreatic cancer. *Current Treatment Options in Oncology*,Vol. 3, pp.449-57.

Lamigeon, C.; Bellier, J.P.; Sacchettoni, S.; Rujano, M. & Jacquemont, B. (2001) Enhanced neuronal protection from oxidative stress by coculture with glutamic acid decarboxylase-expressing astrocytes. *Journal of Neurochem*istry, Vol. 77, pp.598-606.

Lei, Y.H. & Rogers DF (1999) Effects and interactions of opioids on plasma exudation induced by cigarette evaluated by the intraperitoneal bradykinin-evoked pain method in man. *Clinical and Pharmacol ogicalTherapeutics*, Vol.8, pp.521-542.

Lu, Y.; McNearney, T.A.; Lin, W.; Wilson, S.P.; Yeomans, D.C. & Westlund, K.N. (2007). Treatment of inflamed pancreas with enkephalin encoding HSV-1 recombinant vector reduces inflammatory damage and behavioral sequelae. *Molecular Therapy*, Vol.15, No.10, pp.1812-9.

Machelska, H. & Stein, C. (2003) Immune mechanisms of pain and analgesia. Landes Bioscience/Eurekah.com. Georgetown, TX.

Merkord J.; Jonas L.; Weber H.; Kröning G.; Nizze H.; Hennighausen G. (1997) Acute interstitial pancreatitis in rats induced by dibutyltin dichloride (DBTC): pathogenesis and natural course of lesions. *Pancreas*, Vol.15, No. 4, pp.392-401.

Minter, R.M.; Ferry, M.A.; Murday, M.E.; Tannahill, C.L.; Bahjat, F.R.; Oberholzer, C.; Oberholzer ,A.; LaFace, D.; Hutchins, B.; Wen, S.; Shinoda, J.; Copeland, E.M., III, & Moldawer LL (2001) Adenoviral delivery of human and viral IL-10 in murine sepsis. *Journal of Immunology*, Vol.167, pp.1053-1059.

Okuyama, M.; Shibata, T.; Morita, T.; Kitada, M.; Tukahara, Y.; Fukushima, Y.; Ikeda, K.; Fuzita, J. & Shimano T. (2002) A comparison of intraoperative celiac plexus block with pharmacological therapy as a treatment for pain of unresectable pancreatic cancer. *Journal of Hepatobiliary and Pancreatic Surgery*, Vol. 9, pp.372-5.

Papanastassiou, V.; Rampling R.; Fraser M.; Petty R.; Hadley D.; Nicoll J.; Harland J.; Mabbs R.; Brown M (2002) The potential for efficacy of the modified (ICP 34.5(−)) herpes simplex virus HSV1716 following intratumoural injection into human malignant glioma: a proof of principle study, *Gene Therapy, Vol.*9, pp. 398–406.

Pezzilli, R. & Morselli-Labate, A.M. (2009) Alcoholic pancreatitis: pathogenesis, incidence and treatment with special reference to the associated pain. *International Journal of Environmental Research and Public Health*, Vol.6, No.11, pp.2763-82.

Rahim, R.T.; Meissler, J.J.J.; Cowan, A., Rogers, T.J.; Geller, E.B.; Gaughan, J.; Adler, M.W. & Eisenstein, T.K. (2001) Administration of mu-, kappa- or delta2-receptor agonists via osmotic minipumps suppresses murine splenic antibody responses. *International Immunopharmacology*, Vol.1, pp.2001–2009.

Rees, H.; Sluka, K.A.; Westlund, K.N. & Willis, W.D. (1994) Do dorsal root reflexes augment peripheral inflammation? *Neuroreport*, Vol.5, pp.821-824.

Ren, K. & Dubner, R. (1999) Central nervous system plasticity and persistent pain. *Journal of Orofacial Pain*, Vol.13, pp. 155-163.

Romero, A.; Planas, E.; Poveda, R.; Sanchez, S.; Pol, O. & Puig, M.M. (2005) Anti-exudative effects of opioid receptor agonists in a rat model of carrageenan-induced acute inflammation of the paw. *European Journal of Pharmacology*, Vol.511, pp.207-217.

Saeed, R.W.; Stefano, D.B.; Murga, J.D.; Short, T.W.; Qi, F.; Bilfinger, T.V. & Magazine, H.I. (2000) Expression of functional delta opioid receptors in vascular smooth muscle. *International Journal of Molecular Medicine*, Vol.6, pp.673–677.

Salzet, M. (2001) Neuroimmunology of opioids from invertebrates to human. *Neuro Endocrinology Letters, Vol.*22, pp.467-474.

Sassani, J.W.; Zagon, I.S. & McLaughlin, P.J. (May 2003). Opioid growth factor modulation of corneal epithelium: uppers and downers. *Current Eye Research*, Vol.26, No.5, pp. 249–62.

Satoh, T.; Irie, A.; Egawa, S. & Baba, S. (2005) In situ gene therapy for prostate cancer. *Current Gene Therapy*, Vol.5, pp.111-9.

Sawai, H.; Yamamoto, M.; Okada, Y.; Sato, M.; Akamo, Y.; Takeyama, H. & Manabe T. (2001) Alteration of integrins by interleukin-1alpha in human pancreatic cancer cells. *Pancreas, Vol* 23, pp.399-405.

Schmidt, J.; Compton, C.C.; Rattner, D.W.; Lewandrowski, K. & Warshaw, A.L. (1995) Late histopathologic changes and healing in an improved rodent model of acute necrotizing pancreatitis. *Digestion* Vol.56, pp.246-252.

Schmidt, J.; Rattner, D.W.; Lewandrowski, K.; Compton, C.C.; Mandavilli, U.; Knoefel, W.T. & Warshaw, A.L. (1992) A better model of acute pancreatitis for evaluating therapy. *Annals of Surgery*, Vol.215, pp.44-56.

Schafer, M.; Zhou, L. & Stein, C. (1998) Cholecystokinin inhibits peripheral opioid analgesia in inflamed tissue. *Neuroscience,* Vol.82, pp.603-611.

Schmulewitz, N. & Hawes, R. (2003) EUS-guided celiac plexus neurolysis--technique and indication. *Endoscopy*, Vol.35, No.8, pp.S49-53.

Shah, A.C.; Benos, D.; Gillespie, G.Y. & Markert, J.M. (2003) Oncolytic viruese:cliical applications as vectors for the treatment of malignant gliomas. *Journal of Neurooncology,*Vol.65, pp.203-226.

Sluka, K.A.; Jordan, H.H. & Westlund, K.N. (1994) Reduction in joint swelling and hyperalgesia following post-treatment with a non-NMDA glutamate receptor antagonist. *Pain*, Vol.59, pp.95-100.

Sluka, K.A. & Westlund, K.N. (1993) Centrally administered non-NMDA but not NMDA receptor antagonists block peripheral knee joint inflammation. *Pain*, Vol.55, pp.217-225.

Sluka, K.A.; Willis, W.D. & Westlund, K.N. (1993) Joint inflammation and hyperalgesia are reduced by spinal bicuculline. *Neuroreport* Vol.5, pp.109-112.

Sorkin, L.S.; Moore, J.; Boyle, D.L.; Yang, L. & Firestein, G.S. (2003) Regulation of peripheral inflammation by spinal adenosine: role of somatic afferent fibers. *Experimental Neurology*, Vol.184, pp.162-168.

Sparmann, G.; Merkord, J.; Jaschke, A.; Nizze, H.; Jonas, L.; Lohr, M.; Liebe, S. & Emmrich, J. (1997) Pancreatic fibrosis in experimental pancreatitis induced by dibutyltin dichloride. *Gastroenterology,*Vol.112, pp.1664-1672.

Stein, C. (1995) The control of pain in peripheral tissue by opioids. *New England Journal of Medicine*, Vol.332, pp.1685-1690.

Stein, C.; Pflüger, M.; Yassouridis, A.; Hoelzl, J.; Lehrberger, K.; Welte, C. & Hassan, A.H. (1996) No tolerance to peripheral morphine analgesia in presence of opioid expression in inflamed synovia. *Journal of Clinical Investigation*, Vol.98, No.3, pp.793-9.

Steiner, I.; Spivack, J.G.; Deshmane, S.L.; Ace, C.I.; Preston, C.M., & Fraser, N.W. (1990) A herpes simplex virus type 1 mutant containing a nontransinducing Vmw65 protein establishes latent infection in vivo in the absence of viral replication and reactivates efficiently from explanted trigeminal ganglia. *Journal of Virology*, Vol.64, pp.1630-1638.

Taylor, B.K.; Peterson, M.A.; Roderick, R.E.; Tate, J.; Green, P.J.; Levine, J.O. & Basbaum, A.I. (2000) Opioid inhibition of formalin-induced changes in plasma extravasation and local blood flow in rats. *Pain*, Vol.84, pp.263–270.

Thomas, D.L. & Fraser, N.W. (2003) HSV-1 therapy of primary tumors reduces the number of metastases in an immune-competent model of metastatic breast cancer. *Molecular Therapy*, Vol.8, pp.543-51.

Todo, T. (2002) Oncolytic virus therapy using genetically engineered herpes simplex viruses. *Human Cell* Vol.15, pp.151-159.

Toyoizumi, T.; Mick, R.; Abbas, A.E.; Kang, E.H.; Kaiser, L.R. & Molnar-Kimber, K.L. (1999) Combined therapy with chemotherapeutic agents and herpes simplex virus type 1 ICP34.5 mutant (HSV-1716) in human non-small cell lung cancer. *Human Gene Therapy*, Vol.10, pp.3013-3029.

Vardanyan, M. & Rilo, H.L. (2010) Pathogenesis of chronic pancreatitis-induced pain. *Discovery Medicine*, Vol.9, No.47, pp.304-10

Vranken, J.H.; Zuurmond, W.W.; Van Kemenade, F.J. & Dzoljic, M. (2002) Neurohistopathologic findings after a neurolytic celiac plexus block with alcohol in patients with pancreatic cancer pain. *Acta Anaesthesiology Scandinavia*, Vol.46, pp.827-30.

Walker, J.S. (2003) Effect of opioids immune mechanisms of pain and analgesia, In: *Immune mechanisms of pain and analgesia*, H. Machelska and C. Stein (Eds.), Kluwer Academic/Plenum Publishers, Georgetown, TX.

Westlund, K.N. (2000) Visceral nociception, *Current Reviews in Pain*, Vol.4, No.6, pp.478-87.

Westlund, K.N. (2009) Gene therapy for pancreatitis pain. *Gene Therapy*, Vol.16, No.4, pp.483-92a.

Westlund, K.N.; Vera-Portocarrero, L.P.; Zhang, L.; Wei ,J.; Quast, M.J. & Cleeland, C.S. (2009b) fMRI of supraspinal areas after morphine and one week pancreatic inflammation in rats. *Neuroimage*, Vol.44, No.1, pp.23-34.

Wilson, S.P. & Yeomans, D.C. (2000) Genetic therapy for pain management. *Current Reviews in Pain*, Vol.4, pp.445-450.

Wilson, S.P. & Yeomans, D.C. (2002) Virally mediated delivery of enkephalin and other neuropeptide transgenes in experimental pain models. *Annals of the New York Academy of Science*, Vol.971, pp.515-521.

Wilson, S.P.; Yeomans, D.C.; Bender, M.A.; Lu, Y.; Goins, W.F. & Glorioso, J.C. (1999) Antihyperalgesic effects of infection with a preproenkephalin-encoding herpes virus. *Proceedings of the National Academy of Science USA*, Vol.96, pp.3211-3216.

Wolfe, D.; Mata, M. & Fink, D.J. (2009a) A human trial of HSV-mediated gene transfer for the treatment of chronic pain. *Gene Therapy*, Vol.6, No.4, pp.455-60.

Wolfe, D.; Wechuck, J.; Krisky, D.; Mata, M. & Fink, D.J. (2009b) A clinical trial of gene therapy for chronic pain. *Pain Medicine*, Vol.10, No.7, pp.1325-30.

Yang, H.; McNearney, T.A,; Chu, R.; Lu, Y.; Ren, Y.; Yeomans, D.C.; Wilson, S.P. & Westlund, K.N. (2008) Enkephalin-encoding herpes simplex virus-1 decreases inflammation and hotplate sensitivity in a chronic pancreatitis model. *Molecular Pain*, Vol.28, No.4, p.8.

Yeomans, D.C.; Lu, Y.; Laurito, C.E.; Peters, M.C.; Vota-Vellis, G.; Wilson, S.P. & Pappas, G.D. (2006) Recombinant herpes vector-mediated analgesia in a primate model of hyperalgesia. *Molecular Therapy*, Vol.13, No.3, pp.589-97.

Yu Z.; Eisenberg D.P.; Singh B.; Shah J.P.; Fong Y.; Wong R.J. (2004) Treatment of aggressive thyroid cancer with an oncolytic herpes virus. *Int J Cancer*, Vol. 112, pp.525-532.

Zhou L.; Zhang Q.; Stein C.; Schäfer M. (1998) Contribution of opioid receptors on primary afferent versus sympathetic neurons to peripheral opioid analgesia. *J Pharmacol Exp Ther*, Vol. 286, No. 2, pp.1000-1006.

3

Pancreatic Acinar and Island Neogenesis Correlated with Vascular and Matrix Dynamics

Garofita-Olivia Mateescu[1], Mihaela Hincu[2], B. Oprea[1],
Maria Comanescu[3] and Gabriel Cojocaru[1]
[1]U.M.F. Craiova, Histology Department
[2]"Ovidius" University, Constanta, Histology Department
[3]"Victor Babes" Institute, Bucharest, Pathology Department
Romania

1. Introduction

The pancreas is an organ that has a remarkable "plasticity" so that the demarcation between normal and pathological is particularly difficult; it is sometimes difficult to determine whether a change in structure is the cause or effect of pathological conditions.

In these circumstances of an increasing incidence of chronic pancreatitis, the question of regeneration of acinar structures and islands, in the context of known etiopathological conditions is imperative.

The prevalence of chronic pancreatitis in the context of different pathologies is difficult to be determined, varying probably between 0.04% and 5%. This signifies a superposition of the etiology of acute and chronic pancreatitis although it is known that the most frequent etiology of chronic pancreatitis is alcoholism, in middle-age patients[6].

Over 40% from the patients with chronic pancreatitis are predisposed to acute pancreatitis. The evaluation of the general medicine consult and of the laboratory data is necessary for the accuracy of the etiology and pathogeny, being known that the metabolic autoimmune pathology, the anatomical anomalies, the abusive consumption of alcohol also induce hepatic lesions, thus it can be spoken from a hepato-pancreatic lesional complex[11]. In the present paper the etiologic agent prime conductor of the pancreatic lesions is the main concern. That is why we consider indispensable the evaluation of the immunohistochemical markers, of involvement for each matriceal component and pancreatic parenchyma. Thus, the fibrotic replacement of the exocrine pancreatic parenchyma and the appearance of the inflammatory infiltrate are the main features of the chronic pancreatitis.

In this context, it is compulsory to add immunohistochemical results, knowing the importance of some of them either in the collagen forming or in acino-island tissue and matrix recovery.

Therefore we consider extremely important to observe in dynamic the histo-architectural changes of the stroma and parenchyma.

This is why the approach of island neogenesis and not of the acinar neogenesis must be done like a more complex lesion in a mutual interdependence and vascular-stromal induction.

Therefore we consider interesting island neogenesis evaluation in dynamics of various lesions, so the immunohistochemical results are much larger, by a wide use of antibodies, whom target is not only parenchyma neogenesis, but the whole context of lesional chronic pancreatitis. We say this because the study is done on humans and not on experimental models.

We believe that in this case, of the island neogenesis, many factorial etio-pathogenesis, history and family history, therapeutic actions, multiple risk factors (alcohol, smoking, food habits) can create more or less favorable conditions, aspects that can not be extrapolated to the experimental models.

Therefore we can not stop only to identify newly formed islands without assessing the context of lesion, which is why we considered it appropriate to use a wider range of antibodies, covering both parenchyma and vascular-matrix elements.

2. Chronic pancreatitis pathogenic mechanisms

2.1 Toxic-metabolic mechanism

Alcohol is directly toxic to acinar cell through a change in cellular metabolism. Alcohol produces cytoplasmic lipid accumulation within the acinar cells, leading to fatty degeneration, cellular necrosis, and eventual widespread fibrosis.

In alcoholics without chronic pancreatitis, cytoplasmic fat droplets were frequently found in the acinar cells. Alcoholic patients with chronic pancreatitis expressed lesions such as atrophy and fibrosis.

Alcohol produced a stepwise progression from fatty accumulation to fibrosis. The morphological changes of the cellular organites may likewise represent a toxic change in cellular metabolism from alcohol.

Alcohol is metabolized in pancreatic acinar cells through oxidative and non-oxidative pathways[13].

A criticism of this theory is the lack of proof that pancreatic steatosis is a true precursor to fibrosis, rather than a parallel, reversible, alcohol-related lesion[1].

We consider that there is an inter-relation between multiple factors and that alcohol could be the precursor of other pathological events that lead to chronic pancreatic disease.

2.2 Necrosis-fibrosis

Inflammation and necrosis from episodes of acute pancreatitis produces scarring in the peri-ductular areas. This scarring leads to obstruction of the ductules, leading to stasis within the duct and secondarily, stone formation. Severe obstruction results in atrophy and fibrosis. It was suggested that there is a stepwise progression of fibrosis emerging from recurrent episodes of acute pancreatitis[1].

We consider that the necrosis-fibrosis mechanism has to be correlated with the destruction of excreto-secretory elements.

2.3 Pancreatic stellate cells

These cells have long been known to contribute to hepatic fibrosis. Inactive pancreatic stellate cells are triangular, lipid-containing cells predominantly located in the perivascular regions. When activated, they lose their lipid droplets and transform into a fibroblast-like morphologic appearance, migrating to the periacinar areas.

There is ample evidence to suggest that stellate cells play a central role in the deposition of collagen in the early stages of chronic pancreatitis. Pancreatic specimens from patients with chronic pancreatitis exhibit staining for α-smooth muscle actin (present in activated stellate cells) in fibrotic areas of the pancreas.

Our studies showed that the fibrosis begins in extra-lobular spaces by a hyper activity of the stellate cells especially in alcoholic patients which suggest that alcohol and the oxidative stress which it induces form a pathogenic triangle of the necrotic and fibrotic lesions[1].

It is known that the cytokine profile within the pancreas in patients with chronic pancreatitis is distinct from normal pancreas. Pancreatic stellate cells are stimulated by a variety of cytokines which are emitted during the inflammatory phase of acute pancreatitis, this suggesting that recurrent acute pancreatitis could lead to chronic pancreatitis.

2.4 Oxidative stress

The pancreas is exposed to "oxidative stress" through the systemic circulation or through the reflux of bile into the pancreatic duct, leading to inflammation and tissue damage. Oxidative stress may be exacerbated by increased mixed-function oxidase activity, either from high levels of substrate (*e.g.*, fats, diabetics) or inducers (*e.g.*, alcohol and drugs).

Oxidized products are capable of damaging cellular compounds, possibly inducing pancreatic autolysis.

Oxidative stress is involved in the pathway to fibrosis, it has never been proven to *initiate* the disease. Pancreatic acinar cells are capable of metabolizing alcohol without the involvement of Langerhans island. Oxidized products along with cyto-toxines released in the inflammation represent the main aggression factor for the pancreatic acinar cells, favoring necrosis and fibrosis[1].

3. Materials and methods

For our study we used pancreas specimens obtained from patients who died having chronic pancreatitis of various etiology: alcoholism, hepatic cirrhosis, diabetes, etc. For the initial diagnosis classic hematoxylin-eozine and Davenport staining were used to identify pancreatic islands and select the most representative samples for the immunohistochemical study.

We used 10% formaline solution as a fixative because it is suitable for classical stainings as well as for immunohistochemistry, preserving the antigen expression pattern of cells. The volume of the solution was 10 times higher that the volume of the sample.

The samples were fixed 3-4 days depending of their size, and were paraffin-wax processed. The paraffin blocks were cut using the microtome to 5μm thick sections. The sections were harvested on poli-L-lisyne slides in order to have better adherence and to exclude the eventual cross reactions. These sections were stained for different antibodies (Table 1) using the Dako's EnVision detection system, and DAB (3,3'-diaminobenzidine) as chromogen substrate. The nuclei were counterstained using Mayer hematoxylin.

Antibody	Clone	Cod	Antigen retrieval	Dilution
Anti SMA	1A4	M0851 Dako	pH 6 citrate buffer, heat mediated for 11 minutes in the microwave oven	1:100
Anti CD68	IgG1k	M0814 Dako	pH 6 citrate buffer, heat mediated for 11 minutes in the microwave oven	1:100
Anti CD34	QBEnd-10	M 7165 Dako	pH 6 citrate buffer, heat mediated for 11 minutes in the microwave oven	1:50
Anti Cox2	CX229	Cayman Chemical Company	pH 6 citrate buffer, heat mediated for 11 minutes in the microwave oven	1:50

Table 1. Antibodies used for immunohistochemistry

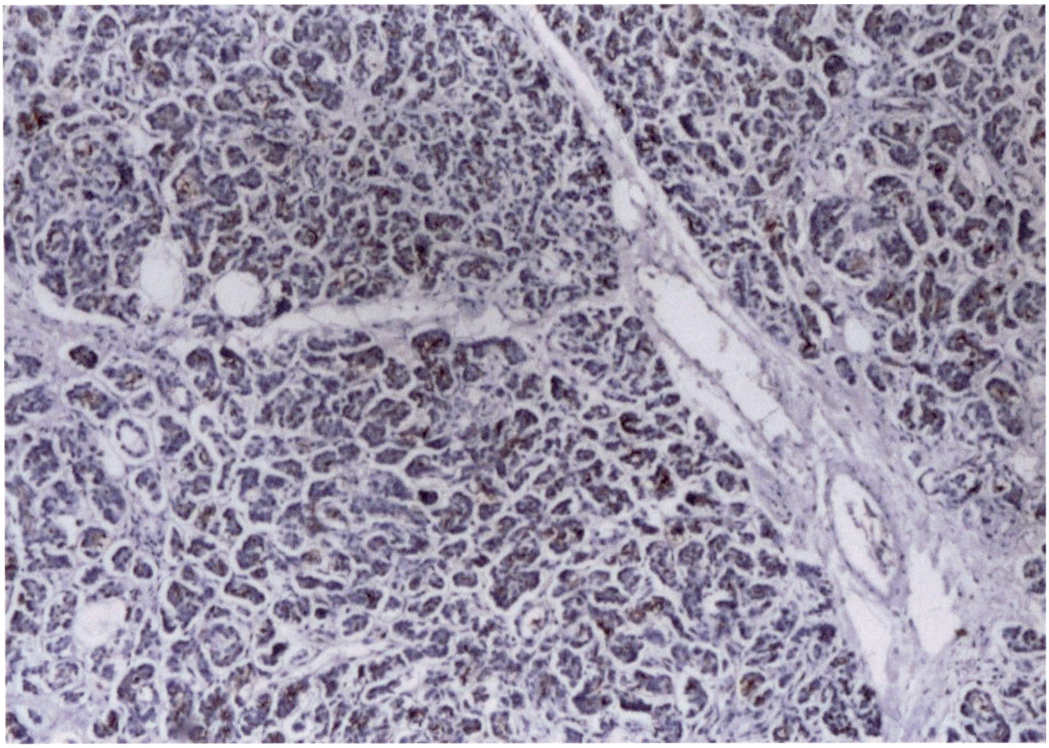

Fig. 1. Cox2 positive immunostaining in acinar cells only

4. Results and discussions

Since inflammatory elements are preserved in vast areas of fibrosis often peri-lesional, we considered interesting to evaluate the COX2[3].

Enzyme inductive COX2 normally absent in cells respond to the action of local and general factors in the evaluation using the immune response by pro-inflammatory role in pancreatitis.

The main features of chronic pancreatitis are involution of exocrine pancreatic parenchyma and endocrine island elements, accompanied by fibril genetics processes and marked inflammatory infiltrate. Therefore, we can not see unilateral these insular and acinar neogenesis, as long as the accompanying inflammatory process may involve prostaglandins.

Inflammatory cells that express COX2, following a specific pancreatic chemo tactics aimed directly the structure, causing necrobiotic damage on one hand, and on the other by phagocytes processes and removing dead cells and cellular debris

It's important to mention that the changes shown in the figure above appear in areas of island neogenesis which in our opinion could be neo-islands. It is possible that the focal positive Cox2 immunostaining to reflect a local immune reactivity to the neo-islets formation. These aspects have been more obvious in patients consuming alcohol comparing to diabetes patients, which suggest the low immune capacity of a diabetic person[8, 19].

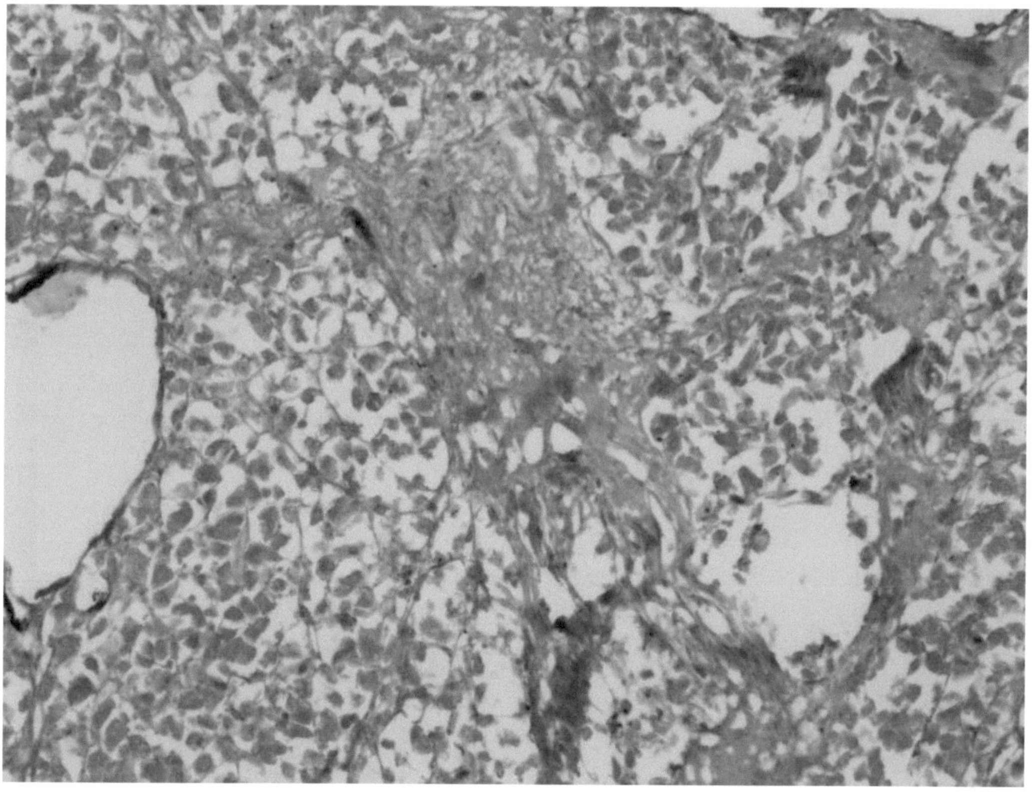

Fig. 2. Focal CD68 immunoreaction in a large area of fibrosis, DAB

So, leukocyte infiltration in chronic pancreatitis is represented by a remarkable percentage of mononuclear cells, which suggests that macrophages have great importance in the inflammatory process. With origin in circulating monocytes, macrophages are activated by certain cytokines and a series of endotoxin, so that their activation can induce phagocytosis. That's why COX 2 inhibitors are accepted therapy of chronic inflammatory lesions[5, 20].

Immunohistochemical response evaluation was approached differently depending on case. For cases diagnosed with early stage chronic pancreatitis imunoreactivity for COX2 was highly positive (62%), while for subjects with diabetes and those diagnosed with advanced chronic pancreatitis was weakly positive (12.7%) or negative response, both ductal and intra-island.

The immunostaining for macrophages (CD68) was reduced compared to Cox2 staining suggesting that the chronic or sub-acute inflammatory reaction is not that much involved in the acino-island regneration.

In advanced chronic pancreatitis, intra and extra-lobular ductal cells were intensely positive for COX-2 compared with islands with variable staining pattern in areas with insulin-positive cells and clinical diagnosis of diabetes[10]. Immunoreactivity was low or absent in people with type II diabetes compared with people consuming alcohol and diabetes type I. These aspects were extremely relevant on the studied samples. Therefore, we consider that a positive COX2 immunoreactivity particularly in intralobular ductal cells enables us to corroborate the involvement of these cellular processes into parenchyma and stroma changes[17,18].

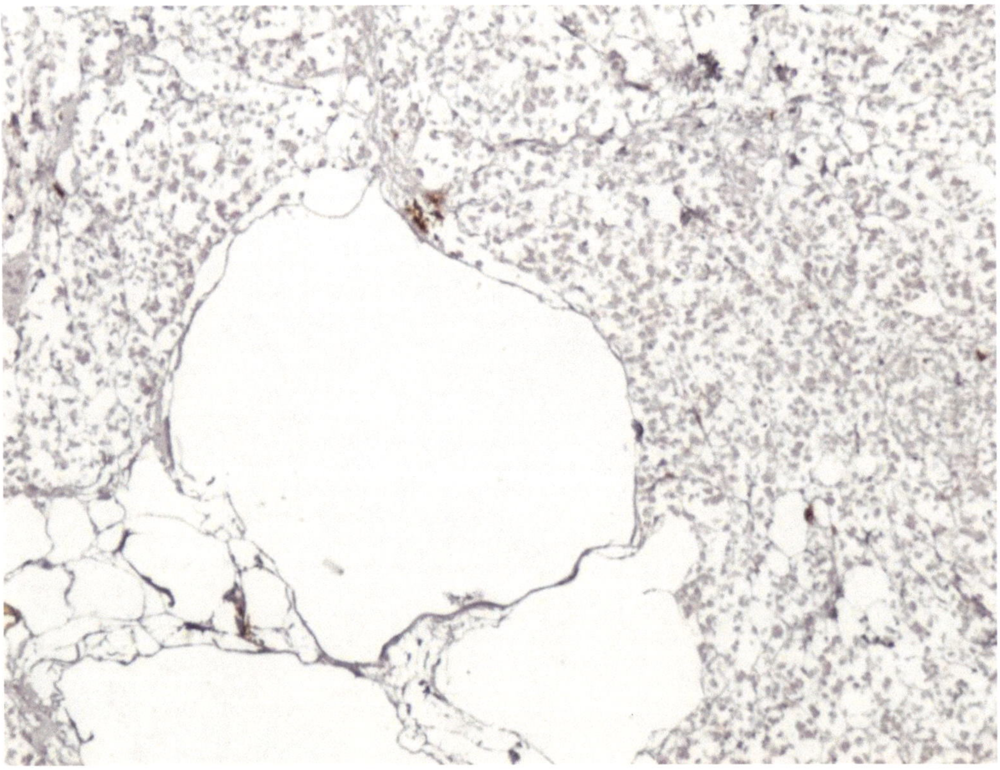

Fig. 3. Focal CD68 immunoreaction near a optic vide areas possible due to focal necrosis, DAB

Due to "pseudo-insular" aspect in areas of parenchyma replacement with remaining acinar structures, the presence of activated macrophages is relevant, stimulating the star-shaped cellularity located at the stromal level, responsible for fibrilogenetics processes in areas with fibrosis[12, 14].

That is why the expression of fibrosis degree with a immunohistochemical response led to the use of matrix metalloproteinases (MMP) involved in regulating fibrilogenesis.

We believe that pancreatic stellate cells (PSC) can act as a central regulator in pancreatic fibrosis in chronic pancreatitis controlling matrix degradation through MMP and TIMP expression, transcriptional regulation process on MMP and TIMP being mediated by cytokines[2].

We consider this issue to be important in chronic early pancreatitis. The immunohistochemical response was highly positive while in diabetics and in subjects diagnosed with pancreatitis due to consume alcohol, immunohistochemical response was weak positive on acinar cells, and even negative in insular cells.

In particular we found in subjects with early-stage chronic pancreatitis, alcohol consumers and non-consumers a binucleation cellularity located in the vicinity of Largerhans islands, and acinar structures with proliferative island aspect, which suggested a possibility of transformation of acinar structures and centro-acinar pseudo-cordonal type items in the drafting of primitive island.

In completing this study, the nestin expression in ductal epithelial cells suggests a possible role in island cells neogenesis. It is believed that the birth of new pancreas endocrine cells occur through mature ductal cell differentiation. That is why there are concepts which suggest that we can not use nestin in human pancreas as a marker of endocrine precursor cells[21].

However, very rarely evidenced in extra-insular cells, with increased nestin expression in neonatal pancreatic islets, we can say, however, it is involved in island neogenesis. This is why it rather indicates a tissue differentiation with diffuse pattern, varying in layout structures with pseudo-insular aspects.

Immunohistochemical nestin positive response was extinguished met both in pancreatic duct cells in appearance and in isolated and small outbreaks in the structures with pseudo-insular aspect, in mature Langerhans island structures, but necrobiotics damages makes difficult to differentiate between different structures.

This reinforces our idea of a possible positivity of tissue remodeling with cell differentiation or functionality exocrine or endocrine-related functionality.

As a result of the vast process of fibrosis processes leading to a reversal of the parenchyma-stroma relationship in favor of the stroma, we were interested in the distribution of collagen IV, a basement membrane major constituent within laminin[13].

Thus, we observed that in subjects with clinically diagnosed early-stage chronic pancreatitis was present a pattern of continuous distribution of collagen IV in basal membrane around ductal cytolysis lesions.

Also, large areas of acinar structures were separated by collagen bands while the remaining islands collagen network sketches pseudo-capsular aspect, so insular cytolysis and modified histo-architecture would be possible by the dual mechanisms.

These issues were particularly characteristic in subjects with advanced chronic pancreatitis. Also, this is very useful especially in differential diagnosis of pancreatic adenocarcinoma where the distribution of collagen IV in basal membrane is discontinuous and irregular or absent around individual cells or groups of tumor cells.

It is known that in normal pancreas, CD 34 positive stromal cells are present predominantly in peri-acinar areas. Isolated CD34 positive cells also were observed in stroma of subjects diagnosed chronic pancreatitis in both advanced and early stage[7,9].

It seems that the presence of significant amounts of CD34 positive stromal cells in primary lesion is characteristic of chronic inflammatory lesions.

In our study, subjects diagnosed with chronic pancreatitis could see an increase in fibrocites CD34 positive. Also, CD34 was positive in vessels in all cases of chronic pancreatitis studied both in diabetics (type I and type II) and drinkers.

This leads us to the idea of involving fibrotic elements which are CD34 positive in a result of stromal remodeling in chronic pancreatitis. Intensively CD34 positive vascular elements were observed in diabetic subjects compared with the rest of the studied

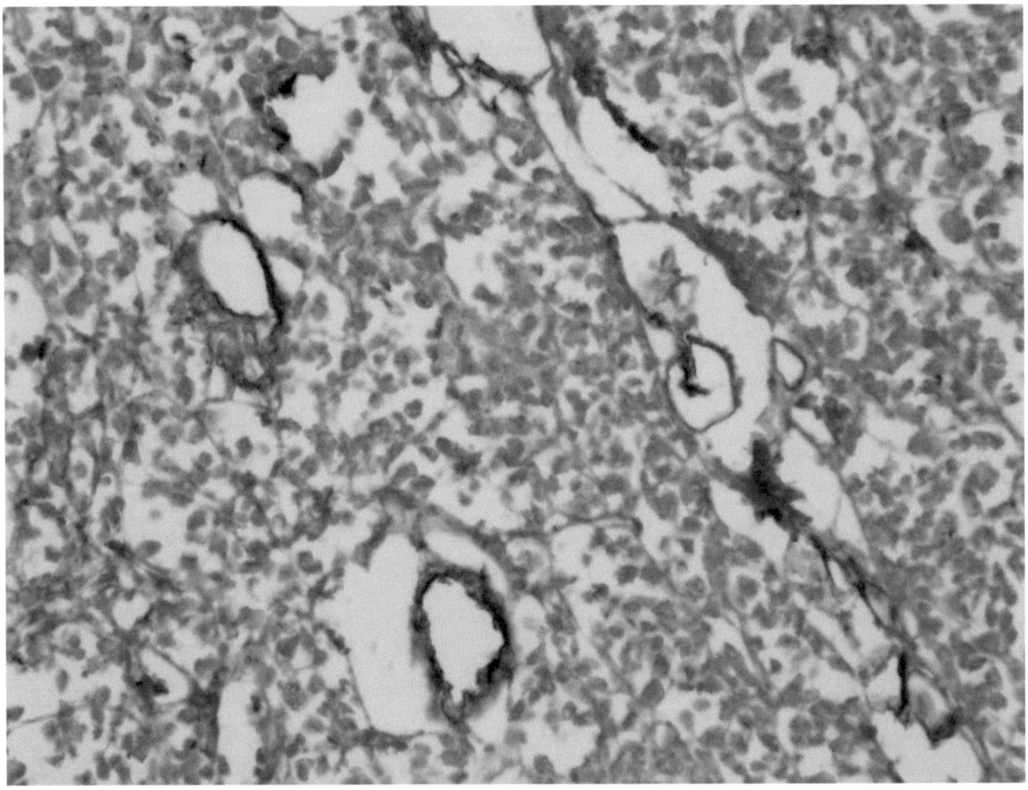

Fig. 4. CD34 immunoreaction in vascular endothelial cells, DAB

Importantly, for an overview of the changes occurring in the matrix and the parenchyma elements, exocrine and endocrine aspects with microscopic positive immunohistochemical markers were mentioned. We consider this relevant because in chronic pancreatitis common lesions can be found but differentiated both at the parenchymal and stromal level. Aspects that we found can be considered to be elements of island neogenesis and are certainly induced by the changes occurring in the overall lesion of chronic pancreatitis. Thus, serous acinar cell nucleus were found in different stages of involution, but the vast majority of nucleus had dispersed chromatin lumps in nucleoplasma or condensed chromatin on nuclear membrane, thereby creating a vacuum optical image space, perinucleolar, something known as "owl eye".

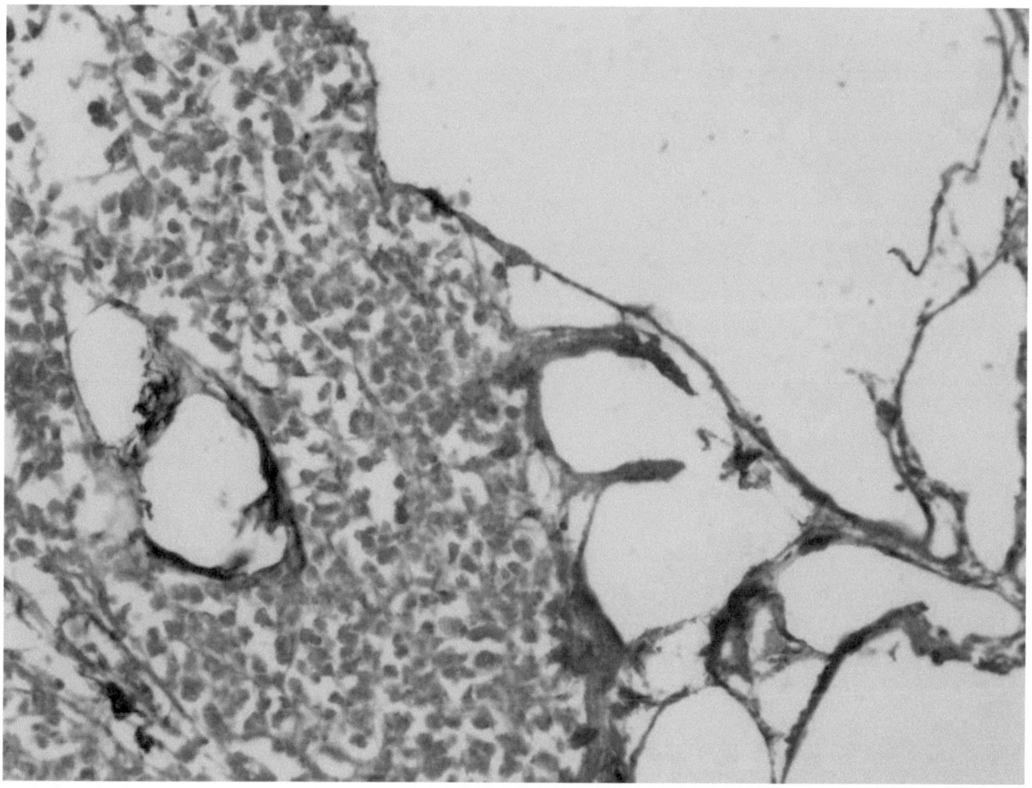

Fig. 5. CD 34 positive in vascular endothelial cells and focal in perivascular cells, DAB

Chronic pancreatitis is characterized by a large number of reactive miofibroblasts to alpha SMA, chronic pancreatitis stromal remodelation being also caused by miofibroblasts, immunoreactive fibroblast-like cells with contractile properties which are considered to be fibroblasts[16, 22]. The TGF-beta has a main role in fibrosis development in liver, but also in pancreas, this suggesting a better research of hepatopathies matter. Many evidences suggest that PSC can be also activated by paracrine profibrogenes cytokines, like trombocytes derivated growth factor and TGF-beta derivated by migratory macrophages. In addition, PSC generate EMC components in return for TGF-beta action, suggesting that the cytokine has an important role in pancreatic fibrogenesis[4, 15, 18].

The apoptosis research, inflammatory injuries, tumoral genesis are controlled by a nuclear transcription factor, NF-kB factor or Kappa B Nuclear Factor. In chronic pancreatitis NF-kB is positive, with intranuclear distribution. Chronic pancreatitis associated hepatic injuries are characterized by hepatocelular apoptosis and necrosis, NF-kB being dependent of liver releasing cytokines and chemakines. Chronic pancreatitis activation can induce hepatic damage through derived Kupfer cells cytokines activation and Fas/Fasl releasing.

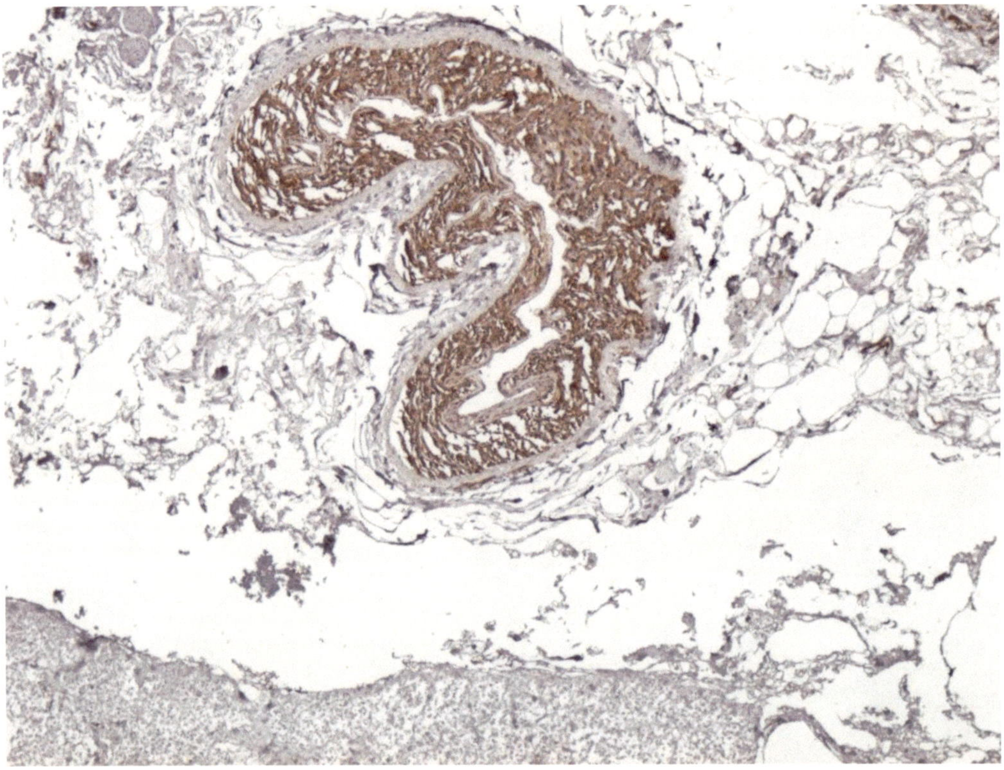

Fig. 6. Anti alpha-SMA staining identifies large vessels with hyaline perivascular deposits, DAB

One aspect we found is that the presence of binucleate cells in the exocrine pancreatic parenchyma. Binucleate cells of polygonal or oval shape present nucleus with condensed chromatin on the nuclear membrane, nucleols and nucleoplasma, obvious tendency to create optically empty spaces. These issues lead us to the possibility of parenchyma neogenesis that we can not exclude taking into account the common embryonic origin of the pancreas with the liver.

Close to capillaries responsible for nutrition of the exocrine parenchyma areas we found the presence of two cell types, some of which were binucleate cells with condensed chromatin on nuclear membrane, with or without obvious nucleoli, and some globular, uninucleate and with nucleoli.

The presence of these cells enables us to believe that they are involved in a possible recovery of pancreatic parenchyma, with the existence of metabolic processes.

Instead, binucleate cellularity was observed in areas of parenchyma completely missing. We noticed the oval binucleate cells with nucleus whose chromatin is cloggy or condensed on the nuclear membrane. Cytoplasm of these cells may present some kind of vacuolization or peri-nuclear argirofile areas in particular.

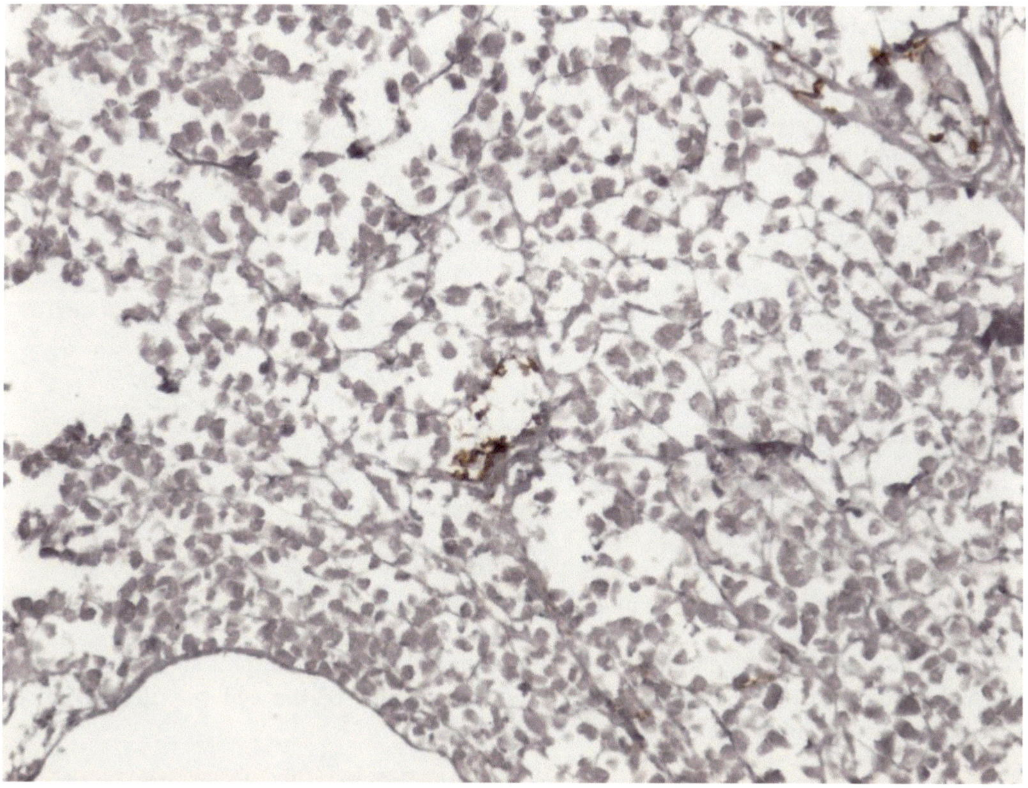

Fig. 7. Anti alpha-SMA staining identifies positive star-shaped cells in parenchyma replacement areas, DAB

Perhaps these cells are involved in pancreatic parenchymal cytological regeneration.

As a result of Davenport staining, we noticed groups of cells containing finely granular and hypo-chromic nuclei, located in the interlobular spaces near the excretory channels. Their appearance is the type of "pseudo-insular" irregular looking with hypo-chromic nuclei and intra-insular argentafine areas.

In the immediate vicinity of these islands we have noted the presence of monoclonal cells with hypo-chromic nucleus fine granular cytoplasm aspect.

These aspects observed in the conjunctive-vascular septas, suggested the hypothesis that, although completely modified, the cyto-architecture of pancreatic parenchyma can regenerate, but without a full morpho-functional reconstruction.

Therefore, we believe that these cell formations are a "primitive form islands."

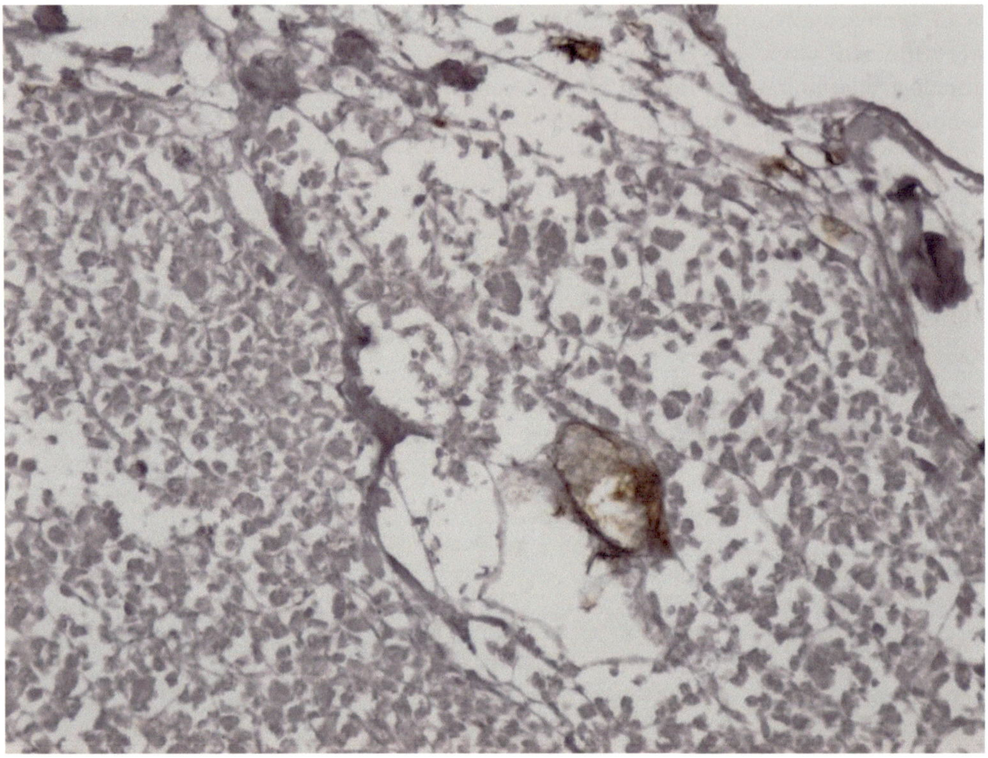

Fig. 8. Alpha-SMA positive staining in middle caliber vessels and intra parenchymatous, DAB

Endocrine parenchymal regeneration issues we noticed in other samples studied, where we found the presence of large cells compared with the rest of the cell population, on the outskirts of Largenhans located islands.

These cells are clearly distinguishable from other island cells, their cell boundaries, appearing not to keep. Cytoplasm of these cells has a fine granular and the nucleus, binucleolat, presents condensed chromatin on the nuclear membrane, giving an embattled appearance.

Besides these large cells, with localization throughout the periphery of the island, we noted the presence of binucleate cells, irregularly shaped. Monoclonal cells with bulky appearance and with binucleate cells were observed mainly in the periphery of Langerhans islands.

That is why the presence of mono-and binucleate cells, large in size compared with the rest of the islet, suggests partial restoration of island celularity.

Pancreatic fibrosis, a characteristic histopathologic appearance of chronic pancreatitis in our study was an active process that, according to some authors, may be reversible in the early stages[13].

Identification and characterization of cells that have fibrilogenesis capacity greatly helped us in the study of pancreatic stroma in chronic pancreatitis. COX-2 played an important proinflammatory role in pancreatitis by regulating prostaglandin synthesis.

As a result of our study we agreed that pancreatic stellar stroma cells mediates fibrosis in chronic pancreatitis with matrix metalloproteinases (MMPS) and tissue inhibitors of metalloproteinases (LONG) -1 and -2 as a modulator of fibrosis

5. Conclusions

We consider that in the pathogenesis of chronic pancreatic disease, multiple factors and theories are involved leading to parenchyma destruction and fibrosis with elements of acino-insular neogenesis.

Immunohistochemical results in the dynamic vascular-stromal and island neogenesis does not clarify the subject. We believe that on the human models we can not have so spectacular results as those experimental models, because the subjects with chronic pancreatitis are exposed to a lot of factors in different evolutionary stages.

6. References

[1] Tyler Stevens, Darwin L. Conwell, Gregory Zuccaro, Pathogenesis of chronic pancreatitis: An Evience Based Review of past theories and recent developments, American Journal of Gastroenterology, 2004; 99: 2256-2270.

[2] Adam J. Ottaviano, Limin Sun, Vijayalakshmi Ananthanarayanan, Hidayatullah G. Munshi - Extracellular Matrix-Mediated Membrane-Type 1 Matrix Metalloproteinase Expression in Pancreatic Ductal Cells Is Regulated by Transforming Growth Factor- βß1 Cancer Res 2006; 66: 7032-7040;

[3] Anirban Maitra, Md, Raheela Ashfaq, Md, Carla R. Gunn, Ayman Rahman, Charles J. Yeo, Md, Taylor A. Sohn, Md, John L. Cameron, Md, Ralph H. Hruban, Md, Robb E. Wilentz, Md - Cyclooxygenase 2 Expression in Pancreatic Adenocarcinoma and Pancreatic Intraepithelial Neoplasia: An Immunohistochemical Analysis With Automated Cellular ImagingAm J Clin Pathol 118(2):194-201, 2002.

[4] Apte M.V., P S Haber, S J Darby, S C Rodgers, G W Mccaughan,M A Korsten, R C Pirola, J S Wilson - Pancreatic stellate cells are activated by proinflammatory cytokines: implications for pancreatic fibrogenesis – Gut., 1999;44:534–541;

[5] Ardeleanu Carmen, Comănescu Violeta, Zaharia B. - Imunohistochimie, ed. Sitech, 1999; 140-146;

[6] Banciu T., Susan L., Jovin G. şi col. – Prevalence of chronic (latent) pancreatitis in hospitalized chronic consumers of alcohol, Rom. J. Med., 1991, Jan – Jun; 29 (1 -2): 49 – 53;

[7] Barth P. J., Ebrahimsade S., Hellinger A., Moll R., Ramaswamy Annette - CD34[+] fibrocytes in neoplastic and inflammatory pancreatic lesions European Society of Pathology Virchows Archiv (Virchows Arch.) ISSN 0945-6317 2002, vol. 440, n°2, pp. 128-133 (24 ref.);

[8] Gray Kd, Simovic Mo, Blackwell Ts, Christman Jw, May Ak, Parman Ks, Chapman Wc, Stain Sc. Activation of nuclear factor kappa B and severe hepatic necrosis may mediate systemic inflammation in choline-deficient/ethionine-supplemented diet-induced pancreatitis. Pancreas. 2006 Oct;33(3):260-7.

[9] Kuroda N, Toi M, Nakayama H, Miyazaki E, Yamamoto M, Hayashi Y, Hiroi M, Enzan H. - The distribution and role of myofibroblasts and CD34 - positive stromal cells in

normal pancreas and various pancreatic lesions. Histol Histopathol. 2004 Jan;19(1):59-67;

[10] Mateescu Garofita, Bold Adriana, Mogoanta L., Busuioc Cristina, PANDURU LAURENTIA - Studiul histologic parenchimo-stromal al pancreasului la persoanele cu diabet zaharat tip 2, Sesiune de Comunicări Stiinţifice, Craiova, 2004;

[11] O'reilly Da, Roberts Jr, Cartmell Mt, Demaine Ag, Kingsnorth An. - Heat shock factor-1 and nuclear factor-kappaB are systemically activated in human acute pancreatitis. JOP. 2006 Mar 9;7(2):174-84.

[12] Palm K, Salin-Nordstrom T, Levesque Mf & Neuman T - Fetal and adult human CNS stem cells have similar molecular characteristics and developmental potential. Developmental Brain Research, 2000, 78 192–195.

[13] Panduru Laurenţia, Bogdan Fl., Mărgăritescu C., Mateescu Garofiţa, - Dinamica stromei pancreatice cronice alcoolice şi nonalcoolice, Sesiune de Comunicări Ştiinţifice, Craiova, 2004;

[14] Phillips Pa, Mccarroll Ja, Park S, Wu Mj, Pirola R, Korsten M, et al. Rat pancreatic stellate cells secrete matrix metalloproteinases: implications for extracellular matrix turnover. Gut 2003; 52:275-82.

[15] Phillips Pa, Wu Mj, Kumar Rk, Doherty E, Mccarroll Ja, Park S, et al. Cell migration: a novel aspect of pancreatic stellate cell biology. Gut 2003; 52:677-82.

[16] Rietze Rl, Valcanis H, Brooker Gf, Thomas T, Voss Ak & Bartlett Pf - Purification of a pluripotent neural stem cell from the adult mouse brain. Nature, 1994. 412 736–739.

[17] Schlosser W, Schlosser S, Ramadani M, Gansauge F, Gansauge S, Beger Hg. - Cyclooxygenase-2 is overexpressed in chronic pancreatitis: Pancreas. 2002 Jul;25(1):26-30.

[18] Seiya Yoshida, Michael Ujiki, Xian-Zhong Ding, Carolyn Pelham, Mark S Talamonti, Richard H Bell, Jr, Woody Denham, Thomas E Adrian - Pancreatic Stellate Cells (PSCs) express Cyclooxygenase-2 (COX-2) and pancreatic cancer stimulates COX-2 in PSCs. Mol Cancer. 2005; 4: 27.

[19] Shi C, Zhao X, Lagergren A, Sigvardsson M, Wang X, Andersson R. - Immune status and inflammatory response differ locally and systemically in severe acute pancreatitis. Scand J Gastroenterol. 2006 Apr;41(4):472-8.

[20] Shimizu K, Kobayashi M, Tahara J, Shiratori K. Cytokines and peroxisome proliferator-activated receptor gamma ligand regulate phagocytosis by pancreatic stellate cells. Gastroenterology 2005; 128:2105-18.

[21] Street C N, J R T Lakey, K Seeberger, L Helms, R V Rajotte, A M J Shapiro, Korbutt G S - Heterogenous expression of nestin in human pancreatic tissue precludes its use as an islet precursor marker. Journal of Endocrinology (2004) 180, 213–225.

[22] Suda K, Fukumura Y, Takase M, Kashiwagi S, Izumi M, Kumasaka T, Suzuki F. Activated perilobular, not periacinar, pancreatic stellate cells contribute to fibrogenesis in chronic alcoholic pancreatitis. Pathol Int 2007; 57:21-5.

Part 2

Diagnosis and Treatment of Chronic Pancreatitis

4

The Role of Endoscopic Ultrasound to Diagnose, Exclude or Stablish the Parenchimal Changes in Chronic Pancreatitis

José Celso Ardengh[1] and Eder Rios Lima-Filho[2]
[1]*Endoscopy Unit, Hospital 9 de Julho, São Paulo,*
[2]*Endoscopy Unit, Division of Surgery and Anatomy,*
Ribeirão Preto School of Medicine, University of São Paulo,
Brazil

1. Introduction

Chronic pancreatitis (CP) can be defined as an inflammatory disease with progressive and irreversible morphological changes (1). There is loss of endocrine and / or exocrine function, with or without pain (2-6). The structure is altered by inflammation, necrosis, fibrosis and loss of exocrine and endocrine elements (5,6).

Alcoholism accounts for 70 to 80% of CP ; 10 to 20% are idiopathic and the remaining 5-10% are caused by hypercalcemia, trauma, hereditary diseases, hyperlipidemia (types I, IV and V) or nutritional causes (tropical pancreatitis) (3, 5, 6).

CP is associated with a mortality rate of approximately 50% within 20 to 25 years after its onset (2,6). About 15 to 20% of patients die due to complications associated with attacks of CP, and most of the remaining deaths are due to trauma, malnutrition, infection or smoking (often associated with alcoholism) (2,6). Very little is known about the actual prevalence or incidence of CP, although estimates indicate an incidence of 3.5 to 4 cases per 100.000 (2,6).

2. Symptomatology

Clinical presentation of CP is characterized by attacks of pain (1). This is intense, localized in the epigastrium, radiating to the back and may also be present in the right or left hypochondria and be associated with nausea and vomiting (1). Usually lasts for hours, although some patients experience continuous pain for days or weeks (3, 5, 6). Along with the destruction of pancreatic tissue there are signs of endocrine pancreatic insufficiency (impaired glucose tolerance, diabetes mellitus) and / or exocrine (steatorrhea) (3, 5, 6).

3. Diagnosis

The diagnosis is based on morphological (abnormalities of pancreatic channels) and functional criteria (pancreatic insufficiency). Although it is easy in advanced forms (Figure 1), in early stages, diagnosis is difficult (7). Ideal diagnostic criteria would be histological (8). However, pancreatic biopsy is susceptible to serious complications, especially in normal or slightly impaired pancreas. In addition, irregular distribution of lesions can lead to diagnostic errors (false-negative) (8,9).

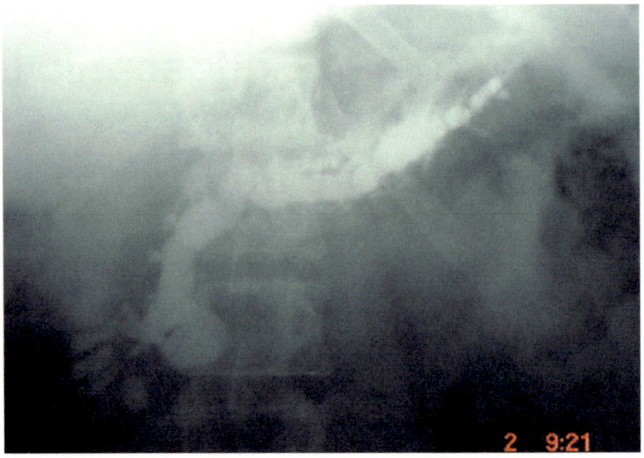

(a)

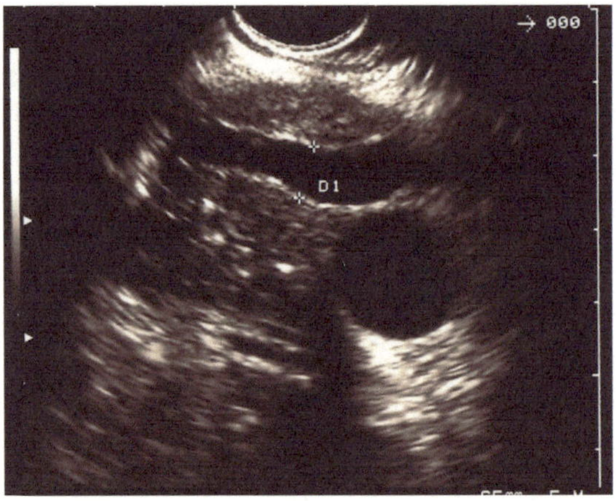

(b)

Fig. 1. Image obtained by wirsungography (a): dilation of MPD and secondary branches. It suggests CP. Echoendoscopic image (b) of the same patient. Besides dilatation of main pancreatic duct (MPD), there are hyperechoic streaks, and hypoechoic areas permeating normal parenchyma.

The development of a technique that could be able to detect early morphological abnormalities and besides that could search for specific cellular or CP biochemical markers in pancreatic juice would represent a significant advance in this field (6,9).

4. Imaging

Similar to AP, US is considered the first exam for patients with suspected CP (7). It shows localized or diffuse increase in pancreatic volume, irregularities and dilations of main pancreatic duct (MPD), or cystic collections adjacent to the gland, and pancreatic calcifications (Figure 2) (2,9-11). Intravenous injection of secretin may be useful in early forms of CP, enhancing discrete changes in MPD caliber (12). Sensitivity and specificity of ultrasound to diagnose CP ranges from 50 to 70% and 80 to 90%, respectively (6, 10, 13).

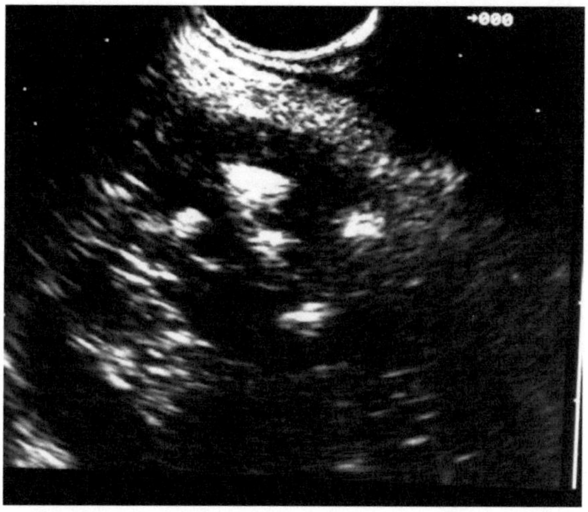

Fig. 2. Echoendoscopic image showing multiple hyperechoic areas with posterior acoustic shadow in a patient with calcifying CP.

A study comparing US, CT and endoscopic retrograde cholangiopancreatography (ERCP) demonstrated that US has a sensitivity of 58% and specificity of 75% to diagnose CP (14). CT is more sensitive and accurate than plain films or US. The suggestive findings of CP include: glandular atrophy, irregularities in pancreatic contours, dilation and irregularities of pancreatic channels with pancreatic calcifications (15). CT is the most sensitive test to detect calcifications and it is still important to search for complications such as pseudocysts. CT sensitivity varies from 74 to 90% and its specificity is over 85% to diagnose CP (2,6). In aforementioned study, CT had a sensitivity of 75% and specificity of 95% (14).

Magnetic resonance imaging (MRI) and magnetic resonance cholangiopancreatography (MRCP) are new non-invasive methods, (no sedation, no contrast, no endoscope insertion). They can obtain images of both parenchyma (MRI) and hepatic and billiary channels (MRCP). They can identify pancreatic atrophy, MPD stenosis or dilation, collateral branches dilation and intracanalicular lesions (16-18).

Our experience is according to literature, and shows that the concordance between MRCP and ERCP varies from 83% to 92% in canalicular dilation, 70% to 92% in canalicular stenosis and 92% to 100% when intracanalicular lesions are present (16, 18, 19). Often, minor abnormalities detectable by ERCP are often undetectable by MRCP and, the rate of false-positive results in canalicular stenosis is high (16,18). Although MRCP is useful to detect moderate and advanced forms of CP, it has a limited value in the early stages (9,18).

Intravenous administration of secretin during MRCP is an alternative to enhance image of MPD in the early stages of CP, as it improves the diagnostic yield (20,21). Image interpretation should be cautious, keeping in mind that artifacts may occur during its reconstruction, leading to a misconception of obstruction, stenosis and stones (21, 22).

ERCP is considered the "gold standard" for diagnosis and treatment of CP (6, 9). Its sensitivity ranges from 74% to 95% and specificity from 90% to 100% (14). A recent study including 202 patients with suspected CP tried to compare the results of ERCP and pancreatic stimulation by secretin- pancreozymin test (TSP), as it is a more sensitive method to assess pancreatic function. The results showed significant correlation between ERCP and TSP, although in 21% of patients, they were discordant and in 15% the results have been contradictory (normal ERCP and abnormal TSP, or vice- versa) (23).

ERCP has some limitations to diagnose CP. Failure in pancreatic channels opacification occurs in 7.5% of cases, particularly when there is an obstruction in the papillary region caused by a stone (9). Invasive nature of ERCP leads to a risk of acute pancreatitis in 5% to 10% of cases, especially in normal or slightly altered pancreas (24). Pancreatography can be normal in 15% of CP and diagnosis is based on clinical course, pancreatic function tests or other imaging methods (6). This occurs more frequently in non-calcified forms of CP (2, 5, 6, 9).

Recently, Tamura et al. (18) compared ERCP to MRI in patients with CP. The authors studied the results of both methods to measure the diameter and characteristics of MPD. The study showed that ERCP tends to overestimate MPD caliber and that MRI is more accurate to define discrete changes in its caliber (18)

5. Echoendoscopy

Echoendoscopy can evaluate in detail all the pancreatic parenchyma as well MPD with no fluoroscopy or contrast (25). Moreover, it is a less invasive method and so, unlike ERCP, the patient has no risk of acute pancreatitis. Echoendoscopic criteria for CP are based on parenchyma and canalicular abnormalities (Table 1) (26,27).

Type of change	Catalano et al.		Sahai et al.	
Parenchyma	Parenchyma	Ductal	Parenchyma	Ductal
Echotexture	Heterogeneous	---	---	---
Focus	Echogenic (1 to 3 mm)	---	Hyperechoic	---
Streaks (interlobular septa)	Hyperechoic	---	Hyperechoic	---
Lobulation	Present	---	Present	---
Pancreatic duct				
Diameter	---	> 3 mm	---	Dilated
Appearence	---	Tortuous	---	Irregular
Hyperechoic focus inside	---	Present	---	---
Hyperechoic wall	---	---	---	Present
Secondary ducts	---	Ectasia	---	Visible
Calcifications and cysts	> 5mm	---	Present	

Table 1. Echoendoscopic criteria for chronic pancreatitis.

US establishes criteria only in severe CP. There are no criteria for mild and moderate CP (28). Figures 3, 4, 5 and 6 show different echoendoscopic degrees of CP. EE has described new imaging criteria to diagnose CP (29).

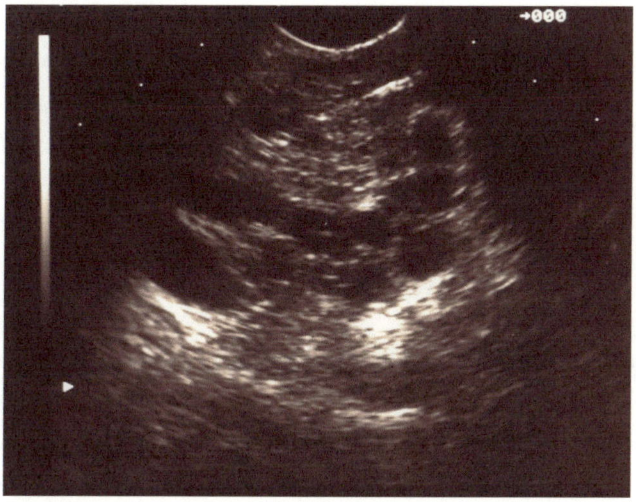

(a)

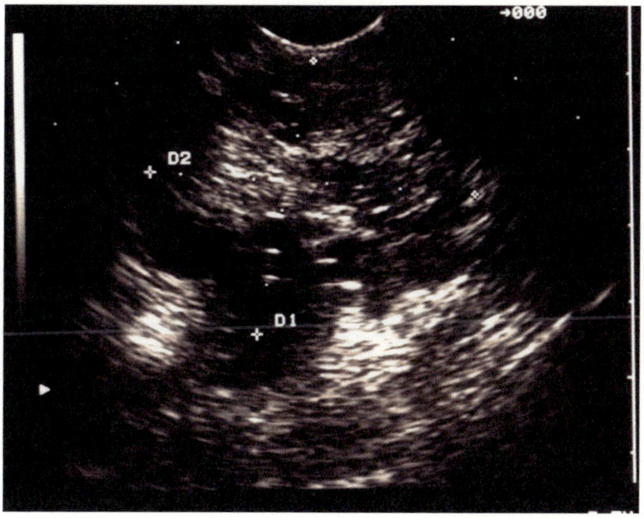

(b)

Fig. 3. Echoendoscopic images in patients with abdominal pain. (a) Hypoechoic areas, intermingled with normal parenchyma and hyperechoic streaks. The aspect remembers a "honeycomb". This aspect suggests early-stage chronic pancreatitis. (b) The same aspect, but more pronounced.

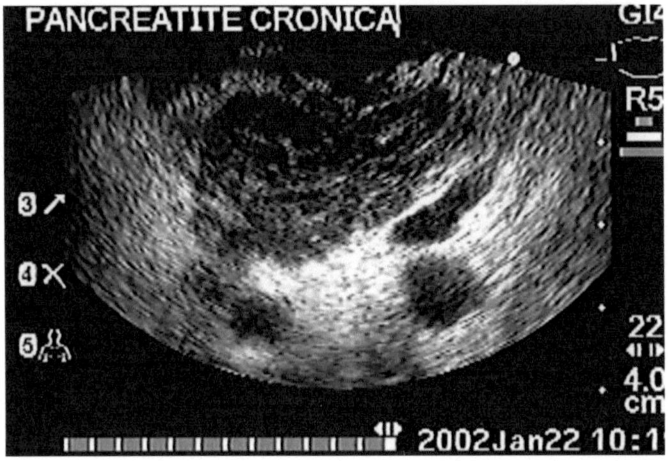

(a)

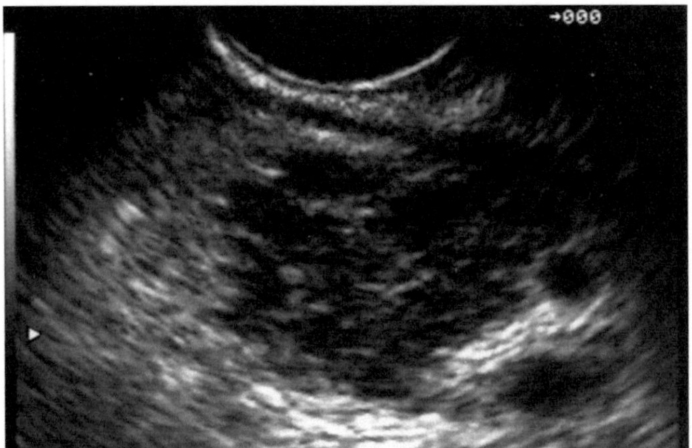

(b)

Fig. 4. Echoendoscopic image of a lobulated pancreatic gland, with hyperechoic striations interspersed with oval hypoechoic areas, and discrete posterior hyperechoic enhancement. This aspect suggests moderate CP.

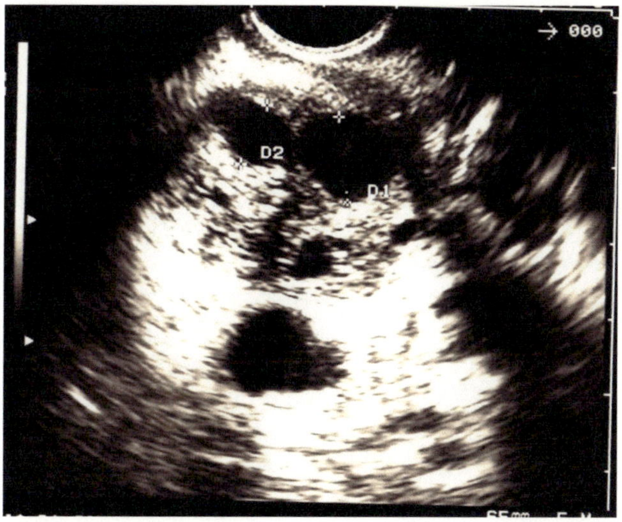

(a)

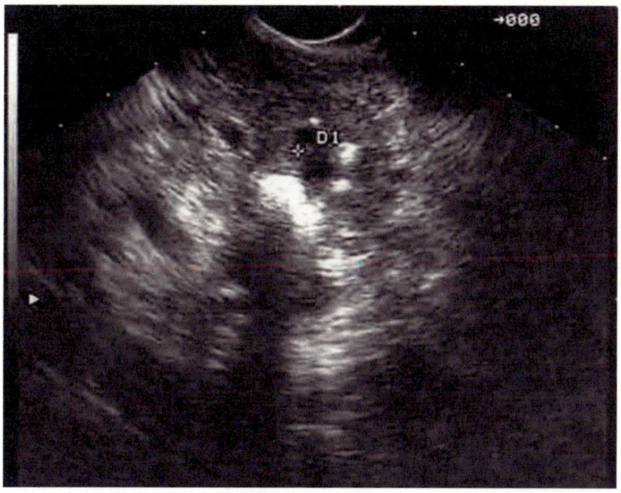

(b)

Fig. 5. Echoendoscopic aspect of calcifying CP. Hyperechoic areas with acoustic shadow and lobular aspect of the gland. (a) dilation of MPD and secondary ducts.

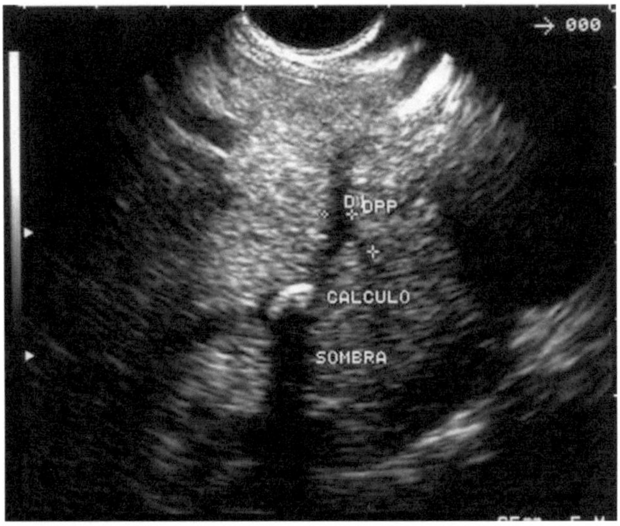

(a)

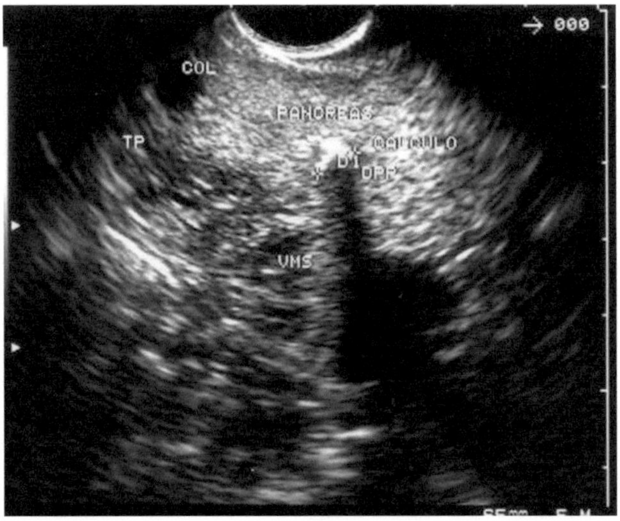

(b)

Fig. 6. Echoendoscopic images showing MPD with a single stone.

6. Echoendoscopy to diagnose early stage chronic pancreatitis

Diagnosis of early stage is a huge challenge. The inability to obtain biopsies makes this presumptive diagnosis difficult. The avaiable diagnostic imaging methods do not offer greater benefits. EE is a promising diagnostic modality and unlike ERCP does not have the same complication rate. Minimal changes in echotexture are difficult to interpret because there is no gold standard (Figure 7).

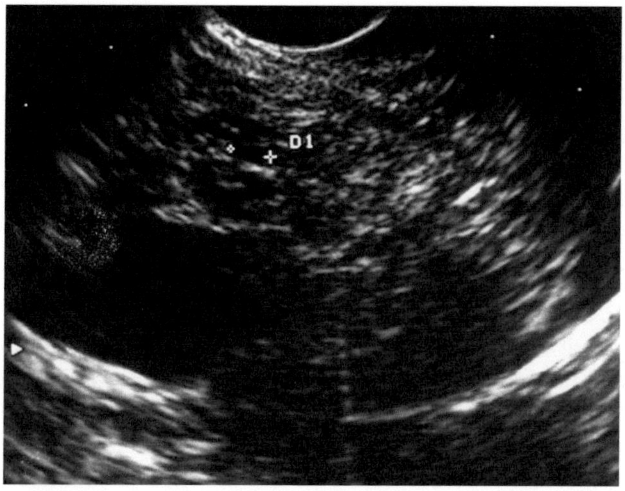

Fig. 7. Echoendoscopic image of pancreas showing parenchymal changes such as: longitudinal hyperechoic streaks, hypoechoic areas, secondary duct dilation and hypoechogenicity of the entire gland.

There is some evidence in the literature suggesting that these early changes may progress to a more advanced disease (30). It is generally accepted that in the absence of all criteria, CP is unlikely, whereas when there is 5 or more of these criteria CP is likely, even when ERCP and pancreatic function tests are normal. Significance of 1-4 criteria is still uncertain, particularly if other diagnostic methods such as ERCP and functional tests are normal (30). In these cases, there is strong evidence of CP, even if these changes detected by EE could not be confirmed by other diagnostic modalitics. A question still remains : How can we improve and understand the abnormalities detected by EE when other tests are normal? The answer can only be obtained from studies with more rigorous methodology.

Yusoff & Sahai (31) prospectively studied 1157 patients. The most important predictive factor for parenchymal abnormalities was alcohol intake, male, clinical suspicion of pancreatic disease and smoking. The authors conclude that many variables can change echoendoscopic aspects and severe abnormalities may be found in asymptomatic individuals. The diagnosis of CP by EE needs to be assessed by clinical, functional and histological tests.

In our department we investigated the meaning of echoendoscopic criteria for MPD and parenchyma abnormalities in patients without suspicion of CP compared to chronic alcoholics (alcohol intake exceeding 80g/ day). Two hundred and twenty-eight patients underwent EE. One hundred and eighty-nine were prospectively studied, using criteria of

Catalano et al. (26) and Sahai et al. (27). Alcoholic patients ($p < 0.001$) showed more abnormalities than nonalcoholic for both scores (parenchyma and MPD). Comparison of ROC curve between the two groups showed a better specificity and sensitivity when the two scores were combined (29). Our results demonstrate a correlation between these signals and the disease, but it is important to emphasize that, in our opinion, echo-guided fine needle aspiration can aid diagnosis and, beyond a shadow of doubts, will be the gold standard for diagnosis of CP, particularly in early phase.

7. Comparison between EE and ERCP

Three studies compared EE to ERCP in order to correlate ultrasonographic and wirsungography signs with severity of CP. In the first, 35 patients with CP were analyzed. Sixty per cent of patients had a history of alcohol intake. There was clear correlation between alcohol abuse and CP ($p < 0.05$) as well with abnormalities of MPD by EE with ERCP ($p < 0.01$). These authors conclude that EE should be the first line method for diagnosis of parenchymal and MPD abnormalities (32).

In the second study, the sensitivity and specificity of EE were 85%. CP is likely because it has a positive predictive value of 85% when more than two criteria (for all CP) or more than six criteria (for moderate and severe forms) are present. Moderate or severe CP is unlikely when less than three criteria are present (negative predictive value> 85%). Independent predictive factors of CP were: calcifications ($p = 0.000001$), history of alcoholism ($p = 0.002$) and total number of criteria ($p = 0.008$) (27).

In the third study, EE and ERCP were compared with a functional (secretin test) and showed a sensitivity and specificity of 84% and 98% to diagnose CP. Although correlation between EE and ERCP is excellent in normal pancreas or in moderate or advanced forms of CP, in early forms it is poor (26). Another study reported sensitivity and specificity of 87% and 89% to diagnose CP (33).

Another study compared the agreement among 11 experienced echoendoscopists to diagnose CP. There was agreement for a definitive diagnosis of CP (Kappa index = 0.45). Agreement was higher for criteria such as ductal dilatation (kappa = 0.6) and lobular aspect (kappa = 0.51). All other parameters showed poor agreement (kappa <0.4). The authors conclude that EE is reliable to diagnose CP, with good correlation among experienced observers (34).

8. Echoendoscopy (EE) alone and associated with fine needle aspiration (FNA-EE)

Hollerbach et al. (8) has recently reported the value of EE with fine needle aspiration puncture (FNAB) to diagnose CP. They concluded that EE is so sensitive and effective as ERCP to detect CP, particularly in early cases. However, echoendoscopic aspects are poor, especially in patients with early disease. EE-FNA is safe and increases negative predictive value of EE. A negative puncture and the absence of echoendoscopic findings of CP could exclude it. It is noteworthy that cytology alone does not increase the specificity of the method, suggesting that tissue collection could impose the use of EE-FNA as a routine to diagnose CP at any stage.

We agree with it.

Patients with CP show another diagnostic difficulty : differencial diagnosis between a real pancreatic mass and a pseudotumour. This diagnosis is relatively difficult to make and an accurate diagnosis could avoid unnecessary surgical treatment (35). Several techniques associated with EE have been described for this purpose. The use of Echo-guided Power Doppler for differential diagnosis showed sensitivity and specificity of 93% and 77% respectively (35). The use of contrast agent (Sonovue) seems to increase sensitivity and specificity rates to 91% compared to EE alone versus 73% and 93% vs. 83%, respectively (36). Echo-guided elastography also contributes for diagnosis, but studies are still preliminary and need further confirmation (35).

EE-FNA has a sensitivity, specificity, positive and negative predictive value and accuracy of 87.5%, 100%, 100%, 98.1% and 98.3% respectively, for differencial diagnosis between inflammatory mass and CP (37).

9. Conclusion

EE has continuously gained importance and has proven to be of clinical value in patients with CP, as it has a low complication rate when compared to ERCP. Some authors indicate EE for examining CP, as it is the imaging method of choice to asses MPD and parenchyma criteria, but there are some limitations. EE has two main limitations that prevent it being the gold standard: the lack of standard criteria for appropriate education and learning (38).

EE is difficult to learn and therefore, teaching has to be standardized. Moreover, a general platform to compare Cambridge criteria is necessary, in order to be accepted as the gold standard to diagnose CP. Except calcifications, the difficulties in assessing some parenchymal criteria depend on differentiation of the natural aging process, the sequelae of pancreatic fibrosis, acute ingestion of alcohol and the advanced stage of CP. Another important point to mention is that the differentiation of hypoechoic (inflammatory x cancer) and cystic lesions (inflammatory x neoplastic) is difficult. In this area, complementary imaging methods have also low sensitivity. Thus there is no doubt that EE has proven to be useful to diagnose CP and its complications (38).

10. References

[1] Kataoka K, Kanemitsu D, Sakagami J, Mitsufuji S, Okanoue T. [Clinical symptoms and diagnostic standards in chronic pancreatitis]. Nippon Naika Gakkai Zasshi 2004;93(1):29-37.

[2] Steer ML, Waxman I, Freedman S. Chronic pancreatitis. N Engl J Med 1995;332(22):1482-90.

[3] Mergener K, Baillie J. Chronic pancreatitis. Lancet 1997;350(9088):1379-85.

[4] Lankisch PG. Progression from acute to chronic pancreatitis: a physician's view. Surg Clin North Am 1999;79(4):815-27, x.

[5] Clain JE, Pearson RK. Diagnosis of chronic pancreatitis. Is a gold standard necessary? Surg Clin North Am 1999;79(4):829-45.

[6] Dimagno MJ, Dimagno EP. Chronic pancreatitis. Curr Opin Gastroenterol 2006;22(5):487-497.

[7] Mayerle J, Stier A, Lerch MM, Heidecke CD. [Chronic pancreatitis. Diagnosis and treatment]. Chirurg 2004;75(7):731-47; quiz 748.
[8] Hollerbach S, Klamann A, Topalidis T, Schmiegel WH. Endoscopic ultrasonography (EUS) and fine-needle aspiration (FNA) cytology for diagnosis of chronic pancreatitis. Endoscopy 2001;33(10):824-31.
[9] Liguory C, Silva MB, de Paulo GA. O Papel da Endoscopia nas Pancreatites Crônicas. In: SOBED, editor. Endoscopia Digestiva. 3a ed. Rio de Janeiro: Medsi Editora Médica e Científica Ltda; 2000.
[10] Niederau C, Grendell JH. Diagnosis of chronic pancreatitis. Gastroenterology 1985;88(6):1973-95.
[11] Bolondi L, Li Bassi S, Gaiani S, Barbara L. Sonography of chronic pancreatitis. Radiol Clin North Am 1989;27(4):815-33.
[12] Glaser J, Mann O, Pausch J. Diagnosis of chronic pancreatitis by means of a sonographic secretin test. Int J Pancreatol 1994;15(3):195-200.
[13] Bastid C, Sahel J, Filho M, Sarles H. Diameter of the main pancreatic duct in chronic calcifying pancreatitis. Measurement by ultrasonography versus pancreatography. Pancreas 1990;5(5):524-7.
[14] Buscail L, Escourrou J, Moreau J, Delvaux M, Louvel D, Lapeyre F, et al. Endoscopic ultrasonography in chronic pancreatitis: a comparative prospective study with conventional ultrasonography, computed tomography, and ERCP. Pancreas 1995;10(3):251-7.
[15] Bearcroft PW, Gimson A, Lomas DJ. Non-invasive cholangio-pancreatography by breath-hold magnetic resonance imaging: preliminary results. Clin Radiol 1997;52(5):345-50.
[16] Takehara Y, Ichijo K, Tooyama N, Kodaira N, Yamamoto H, Tatami M, et al. Breath-hold MR cholangiopancreatography with a long-echo-train fast spin-echo sequence and a surface coil in chronic pancreatitis. Radiology 1994;192(1):73-8.
[17] Cardone G, Di Girolamo M, Messina A, Chichiarelli A, Innacoli M, Di Cesare E, et al. [Magnetic resonance in the study of inflammatory diseases of the pancreas]. Radiol Med (Torino) 1995;90(1-2):62-9.
[18] Tamura R, Ishibashi T, Takahashi S. Chronic pancreatitis: MRCP versus ERCP for quantitative caliber measurement and qualitative evaluation. Radiology 2006;238(3):920-8.
[19] Szejnfeld J, Nakao FS, Araújo I, DIppolito G, Ferrari AP. MRCP and ERCP: a comparison in 45 patients. HPB 1999;1(2):61-64.
[20] Nicaise N, Pellet O, Metens T, Deviere J, Braude P, Struyven J, et al. Magnetic resonance cholangiopancreatography: interest of IV secretin administration in the evaluation of pancreatic ducts. Eur Radiol 1998;8(1):16-22.
[21] Merkle EM, Baillie J. Exocrine pancreatic function: evaluation with MR imaging before and after secretin stimulation. Am J Gastroenterol 2006;101(1):137-8.
[22] Yamaguchi K, Chijiwa K, Shimizu S, Yokohata K, Morisaki T, Tanaka M. Comparison of endoscopic retrograde and magnetic resonance cholangiopancreatography in the surgical diagnosis of pancreatic diseases. Am J Surg 1998;175(3):203-8.
[23] Lankisch PG, Seidensticker F, Otto J, Lubbers H, Mahlke R, Stockmann F, et al. Secretin-pancreozymin test (SPT) and endoscopic retrograde cholangiopancreatography

(ERCP): both are necessary for diagnosing or excluding chronic pancreatitis. Pancreas 1996;12(2):149-52.

[24] Cotton PB, Lehman G, Vennes J, Geenen JE, Russell RC, Meyers WC, et al. Endoscopic sphincterotomy complications and their management: an attempt at consensus. Gastrointest Endosc 1991;37(3):383-93.

[25] Ardengh JC, Pauphilet C, Ganc AJ, Colaiacovo W. Endoscopic ultrasonography of the pancreas: technical aspects. GED 1994;13(2):61-68.

[26] Catalano MF, Lahoti S, Geenen JE, Hogan WJ. Prospective evaluation of endoscopic ultrasonography, endoscopic retrograde pancreatography, and secretin test in the diagnosis of chronic pancreatitis. Gastrointest Endosc 1998;48(1):11-7.

[27] Sahai AV, Zimmerman M, Aabakken L, Tarnasky PR, Cunningham JT, van Velse A, et al. Prospective assessment of the ability of endoscopic ultrasound to diagnose, exclude, or establish the severity of chronic pancreatitis found by endoscopic retrograde cholangiopancreatography. Gastrointest Endosc 1998;48(1):18-25.

[28] Irisawa A, Mishra G, Hernandez LV, Bhutani MS. Quantitative analysis of endosonographic parenchymal echogenicity in patients with chronic pancreatitis. J Gastroenterol Hepatol 2004;19(10):1199-205.

[29] Thuler FP, Costa PP, Paulo GA, Nakao FS, Ardengh JC, Ferrari AP. Endoscopic ultrasonography and alcoholic patients: can one predict early pancreatic tissue abnormalities? Jop 2005;6(6):568-74.

[30] Raimondo M, Wallace MB. Diagnosis of early chronic pancreatitis by endoscopic ultrasound. Are we there yet? Jop 2004;5(1):1-7.

[31] Yusoff IF, Sahai AV. A prospective, quantitative assessment of the effect of ethanol and other variables on the endosonographic appearance of the pancreas. Clin Gastroenterol Hepatol 2004;2(5):405-9.

[32] Alempijevic T, Kovacevic N, Duranovic S, Krstic M, Ugljesic M. [Correlation between findings of echosonography and endoscopic retrograde cholangiopancreatography examination in chronic pancreatitis patients]. Vojnosanit Pregl 2005;62(11):821-5.

[33] Wiersema MJ, Hawes RH, Lehman GA, Kochman ML, Sherman S, Kopecky KK. Prospective evaluation of endoscopic ultrasonography and endoscopic retrograde cholangiopancreatography in patients with chronic abdominal pain of suspected pancreatic origin. Endoscopy 1993;25(9):555-64.

[34] Wallace MB, Hawes RH, Durkalski V, Chak A, Mallery S, Catalano MF, et al. The reliability of EUS for the diagnosis of chronic pancreatitis: interobserver agreement among experienced endosonographers. Gastrointest Endosc 2001;53(3):294-9.

[35] Saftoiu A, Popescu C, Cazacu S, Dumitrescu D, Georgescu CV, Popescu M, et al. Power Doppler endoscopic ultrasonography for the differential diagnosis between pancreatic cancer and pseudotumoral chronic pancreatitis. J Ultrasound Med 2006;25(3):363-72.

[36] Hocke M, Schulze E, Gottschalk P, Topalidis T, Dietrich CF. Contrast-enhanced endoscopic ultrasound in discrimination between focal pancreatitis and pancreatic cancer. World J Gastroenterol 2006;12(2):246-50.

[37] Ardengh JC, Paulo GA, Cury MS, Hervoso CM, Ornellas LC, Lima LFP, et al. The role of endoscopic ultrasound (EUS) with fine needle aspiration (EUS-FNA) in the differential diagnosis of focal chronic pancreatitis (FCP) and pancreatic adenocarcinoma (PAC). Gastrointest Endosc 2005;61(5):AB270.

[38] Jenssen C, Dietrich CF. [Endoscopic ultrasound in chronic pancreatitis]. Z Gastroenterol 2005;43(8):737-49.

5

Endoscopic Treatment in Chronic Pancreatitis

Yue Sun Cheung and Paul Bo-San Lai
Division of Hepato-biliary and Pancreatic Surgery, Department of Surgery, The Chinese University of Hong Kong, Honk Kong, China

1. Introduction

Chronic pancreatitis can give rise to relapsing episodic or persistent upper abdominal pain (Frulloni et al., 2010). Apart from the derangement of endocrine and exocrine functions, it can cause local complications such as pancreatic ductal stenosis, formation of intraductal stones and development of pseudocysts (Strobel et al., 2009). Management of these complications can be challenging in some patients. Various surgical drainage and resection procedures had been described with successful results (Strobel et al., 2009) but they were technically demanding and carried significant morbidities (Schnelldorfer et al., 2007). With the advancement in endoscopic treatments and novel techniques, some of the conventional open procedures have been replaced by endoscopic or minimally invasive techniques. In this chapter, we reviewed various endoscopic procedures available in treating patients with chronic pancreatitis, namely endoscopic sphincterotomy, stricture dilatation, stenting, stone extraction, endoscopic ultrasound-guided pseudocyst drainage and celiac plexus block. The indications, techniques and efficacy of endoscopic treatments were discussed in this chapter.

2. Indications of endoscopic treatment

Endoscopic treatment can be applied to different pathologic processes associated with chronic pancreatitis. These processes include pancreatic ductal strictures, stones and pancreatic pseudocyst formation (Sherman & Lehman, 1998). These processes can lead to ductal obstruction and parenchymal hypertension, resulting in upper abdominal pain (Strobel et al., 2009). Restoration of the drainage of the main pancreatic duct by a combination of sphincterotomy, stricture dilatation, stone extraction and stent placement are indicated in symptomatic patients with these pathologies (Strobel et al., 2009).

Apart from pain, chronic pancreatitis might also cause pseudocyst formation, leading to abscess, ascites and pleural effusion secondary to rupture and occasionally pseudoaneurysm formation. The formation of pseudoaneurysm could in turn lead to massive gastrointestinal tract bleeding or interperitoneal haemorrhage (Lai et al., 1997). Therefore, drainage of pseudocyst is another common indication for endoscopic treatment.

Recently, pancreatic neuritis secondary to inflammatory infiltration and hypertrophy of pancreatic nerves was proposed as the alternative mechanism causing abdominal pain in chronic pancreatitis (Strobel et al., 2009). Endoscopic ultrasound-guided celiac plexus block had been employed safely for pain relief in chronic pancreatitis with minimal complication (Avula & Sherman, 2010; Puli SR et al., 2009).

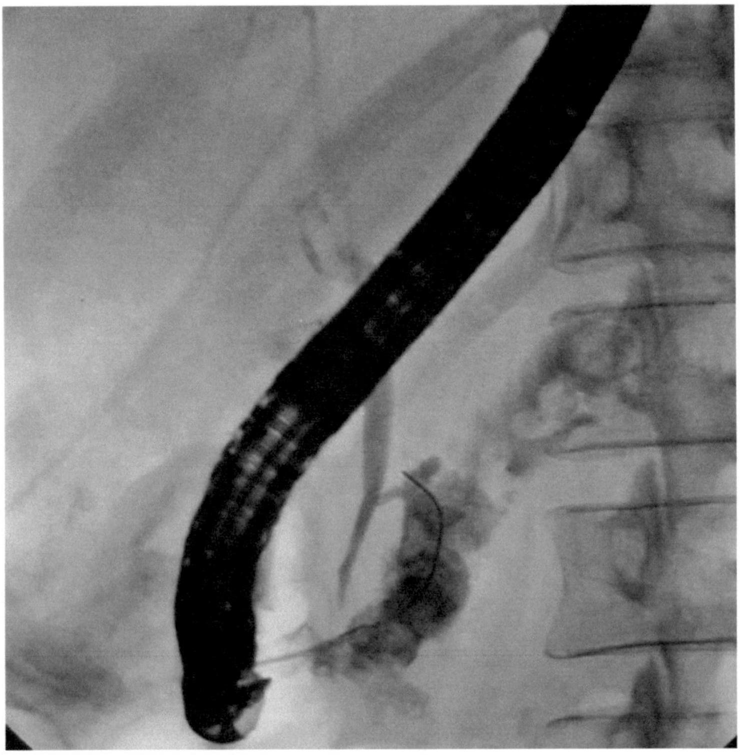

Fig. 1. Multiple pancreatic ductal stones with ductal dilatation on ERCP.

Although indications of endoscopic therapy to chronic pancreatitis might extend with more data coming up, it has little role in asymptomatic main pancreatic duct dilatation at the moment. There has been no data to suggest the restoration of the pancreatic outflow can delay the process of pancreatic parenchymal atrophy or improve the endocrine and exocrine function of pancreas (Frulloni et al., 2010).

3. Techniques of endoscopic treatment

With the advance in technology and improvement in endoscopic skills, various endoscopic therapies in chronic pancreaittis are made possible. The following sections described the common techniques used in chronic pancreaitits.

3.1 Endoscopic sphincterotomy

Endoscopic sphincterotomy can be performed by either standard pull-type sphincterotomy after wire-guided cannulation or pre-cut on pancreatic stent (Buscaglia & Kalloo, 2007). However, unlike biliary sphincterotomy, the direction of pancreatic sphincterotomy should be directed towards the 1 to 2 o'clock position of the papillary orifice. An incision of 5 to 10mm in length is usually made with the pure cutting current, so that damage to the pancreas and subsequent stenosis of papilla can be avoided. A pancreatic stent is usually put in temporarily to prevent ductal obstruction by post-sphincterotomy edema (Buscaglia & Kalloo, 2007).

Occasionally pathology at the minor papilla such as pancreatic divisum, can be a cause of chronic pancreatitis (Tarnasky et al., 1997). Minor papillotomy, dividing only the mucosal mound rather than true sphincterotomy, can be performed to achieve decompression of the dorsal duct (Buscaglia & Kalloo, 2007). A soft tip 0.035 inch hydrophilic guidewire is generally used for wire-guided cannulation. After deep cannulation achieved, standard pull-type sphincterotomy can be performed, directing along the course of the dorsal duct, usually at 11 o'clock position (Buscaglia & Kalloo, 2007).

Endoscopic sphincterotomy can also be performed as the primary treatment for conditions leading to chronic pancreatitis, e.g. sphincter of Oddi dysfunction. It is, however, more commonly used to gain access to the pancreatic duct and facilitate further endoscopic treatment as described in later section.

3.2 Pancreatic ductal dilatation and stenting

Patients with focal main pancreatic duct stricture at the head or body can be managed by dilatation and stenting, usually after pancreatic sphincterotomy. A guidewire can be passed proximal to the stricture site, over which graduated dilating catheter or hydrostatic balloon dilator can be used for stricture dilatation. Since these strictures from chronic pancreatitis are very fibrotic, simple dilatation alone usually does not give long term response (Yoo & Lehman, 2009). Endoscopic stents are therefore placed across the strictures to adequately expand the lumen to achieve a good flow of pancreatic juice even after the stent is removed. Different sizes of stents are used for different purpose, but they should not be larger than the diameter of the distal duct. In general, stents for pancreatitis prophylaxis are usually 3-5 Fr in size, whereas single or multiple stents up to 7 to 10 Fr might be necessary after stricture dilatation (Yoo & Lehman, 2009). The optimal duration to leave a stent in-situ is not known

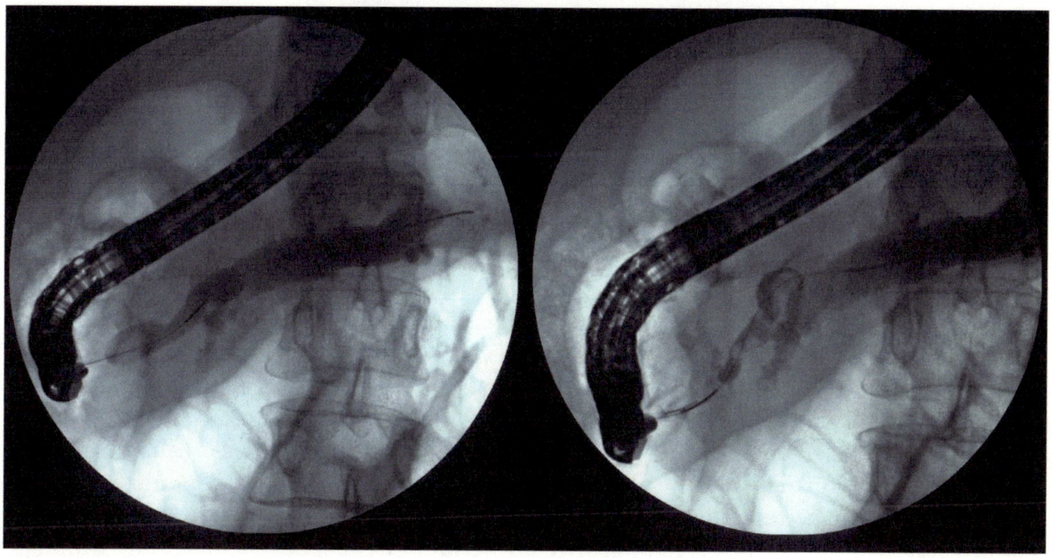

Fig. 2. Pancreatic ductal stricture dilatation with balloon dilator.

(Sherman & Lehman, 1998). It can be left till symptoms reappears or can be exchanged at 3-monthly interval (Yoo & Lehman, 2009). In patients with dominant pancreatic duct strictures, the technical success rate up to 91% had been reported but only 62% of these patients had symptoms improved. The morbidity and mortality rate reported were 18% and 1% respectively (Yoo & Lehman, 2009).

3.3 Extraction of pancreatic ductal stones

Removal of pancreatic ductal stones usually requires a pancreatic sphincterotomy to facilitate access to the duct. In cases where strictures distal to the stones are present, dilatation with catheters or hydrostatic balloons is also required. Balloons and baskets are common accessories for stone retrieval and in difficult cases, such as bending across a tortuous duct, over-the-wire accessories might be necessary (Sherman & Lehman, 1998). For very big and hard stones, lithotripsy either using laser or electrohydrolic lithotripsy (EHL) or extra-corporeal shock wave lithotripsy (ESWL) would frequently be necessary.

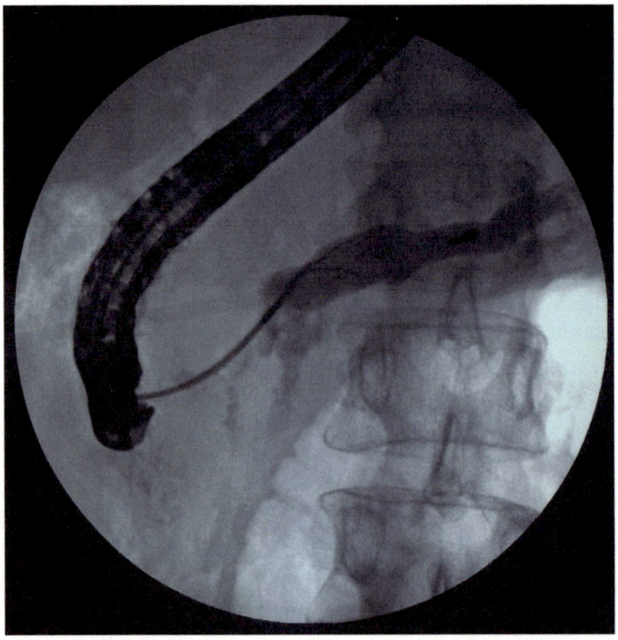

Fig. 3. Pancreatic duct stone removed with basket.

For laser or electrohydrolic lithotripsy, a small caliber through-the-scope pancreatoscope is needed to guide the lithotripsy under direct vision. The pancreatoscope can be passed down the duodenoscope over guidewire to gain access to the pancreatic duct (Howell et al., 1999). After visualization of the stone, the EHL probe or laser fibre is passed down the channel of the pancreatoscope (Howell et al., 1999; Hirai et al., 2004). In case of EHL, lithotripsy is performed with saline lavage to optimize energy penetration. Stone fragments can then be removed by basket or lavage over balloon catheter. A stent without forward flap is usually placed temporarily at the end of procedure to facilitate drainage (Howell et al., 1999).

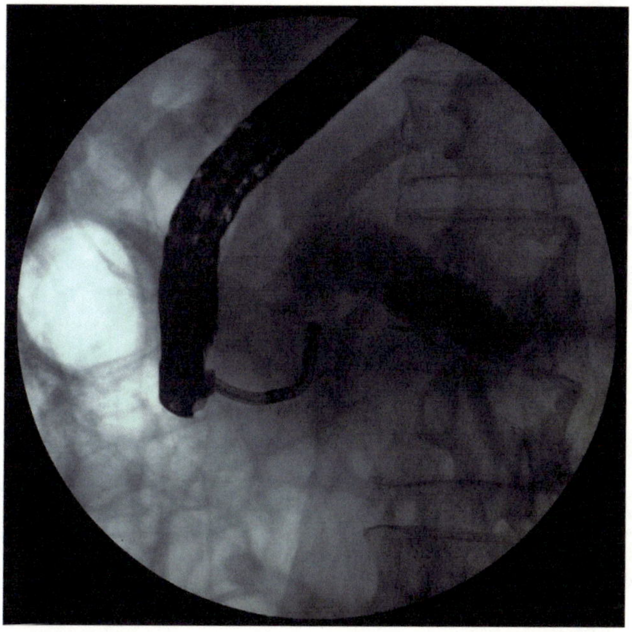

Fig. 4. Pancreatoscope passed down through standard duodenoscope to visualize the pancreatic duct lumen.

3.4 Combined endoscopy and extracorporal shockwave lithotripsy

Extracorporeal shock wave lithotripsy (ESWL) is another adjunct in the endoscopic treatment of pancreatic duct stones (Lawrence et al., 2010). It can fragment the stones and reduce stone burden, thus facilitating endoscopic clearance of the pancreatic duct. Endoscopic sphincterotomy is usually performed before ESWL. Pancreatic duct stones can be localized either by fluoroscopy or ultrasonography during lithotripsy. Contrast instillation through a nasopancreatic drain could sometimes help with the localization of radiolucent stone (Choi & Kim, 2006). Occasionally the nasopancreatic drain can also be used for saline irrigation (Costamagna et al., 1997) and obtain follow-up pancreatograms after ESWL. If pancreatic ductal strictures are present, dilatation and stenting might be performed to facilitate ductal clearance and decompression after stones fragmentation (Choi & Kim, 2006).

3.5 Drainage of pancreatic pseudocyst

Endoscopic drainage of pseudocyst involved the creation of communication between the pseudocyst and gastrointestinal lumen, so that the cyst content can be drained internally (Sherman & Lehman, 1998). The access to the pseudocyst can be guided by means of endoscopic ultrasound (EUS). This facilitate transmural needle placement even when no bulge can be seen through the endoscope and avoid puncturing the vessels on gastroduodenal wall.

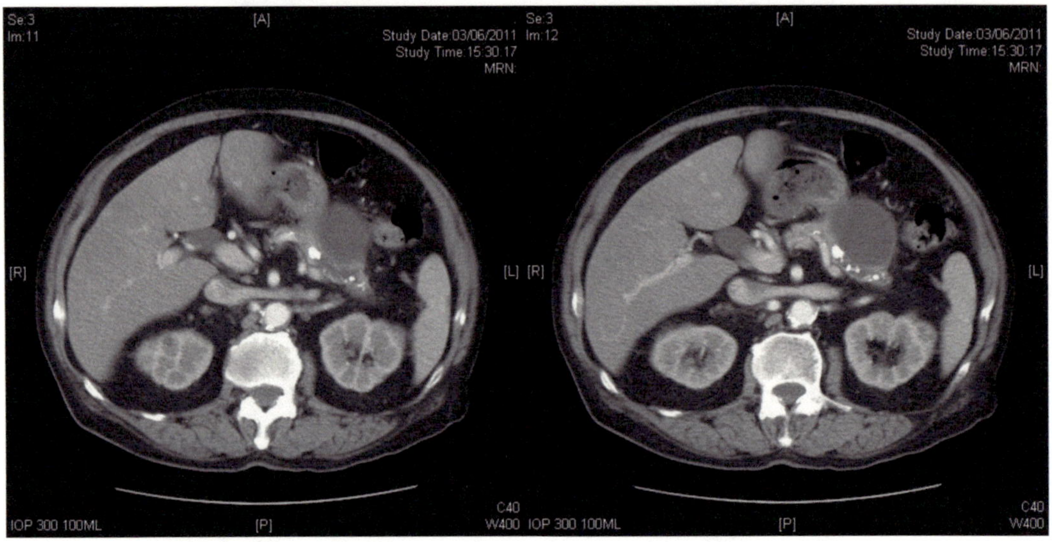

Fig. 5. Computed tomography showing pseudocyst near the tail of pancreas with mild pancreatic duct dilatation and stones proximal to the cyst.

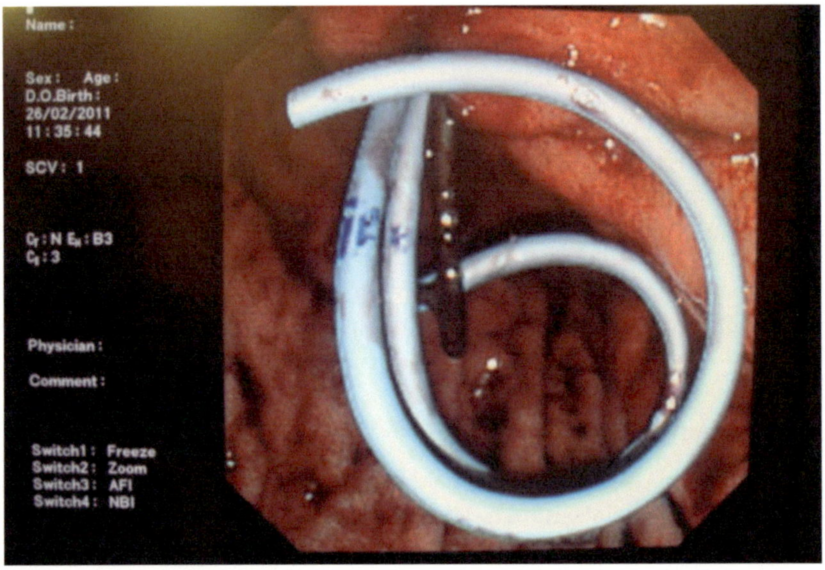

Fig. 6. Endoscopic view of plastic stent and double pigtail catheters inserted under endoscopic ultrasound guidance to form a cystogastrostomy.

The pseudocyst is punctured under the guidance of a linear echoendoscope. A guidewire is passed into the cyst under fluoroscopic control to form at least 2 loops. The cystogastrostomy or cystoduodenostomy is then dilated with balloon catheter to 6-8mm size, follow which a double pigtail stent will be inserted over the wire to establish the drainage. Second or multiple stents will then be inserted under endoscopic and fluoroscopic guidance by recannulation of the pseudocysts (Seewald et al., 2009). In case of abscess or debris are present inside the pseudocyst, saline irrigation and aspiration of the cyst content can be achieved through a nasocystic catheter instead of internal stent.

As recannulation of the pseudocyst can sometimes be cumbersome, some endoscopists advocated the use of "double-wire" technique, in which 2 wires were inserted into the pseudocyst through a double lumen catheter after the pseudocyst is punctured. Simultaneous stents or nasocystic catheters insertion can then be performed under fluoroscopic guidance over the 2 wires in place. (Itoi et al., 2009)

Complications of EUS-guided drainage include bleeding, perforation and infection. Coagulopathy has to be corrected and prophylactic antibotics should be given before the procedure. Only pseudocyst with mature wall and within 1cm from gastrointestinal lumen should be considered for endoscopic drainage (Seewald et al., 2009).

Although EUS-guided drainage is a promising technique for decompression of pesudocyst in chronic pancreatitis, case selection is very important for success. Technical success rate, defined as the feasibility of access and drain insertion to the cystic fluid (Seewald et al., 2009), ranged from 92% to 100%. However, up to 23 % of pseudocyst recurred during a median follow-up period of 22 months (Binmoeller et al., 1995), giving a long term success rate of 65% to 81% (Aghdassi et al., 2008). In case of fail endoscopic treatment, unfavourable cyst location, such as far from the gastrointestinal lumen, or if neoplasm cannot be excluded, surgery is still the standard procedure of choice (Baillie 2004). Surgical drainage procedures can be in form of cysto-gastrostostomy or cysto-jejunostomy depending on site of the cyst. For pseudocyst masquerading cystic neoplasm, distal pancreatectomy or pancreatoduodenectomy should be advised (Cheung et al., 2008).

3.6 Endoscopic ultrasound-guided celiac plexus block

Celiac plexus is located at T12 to L1 level near the take off of celiac trunk adjacent to the aorta. It is a network of ganglia and nerves that lie on both side of the aorta. It contains sympathetic and parasympathetic fibres transmitting signals to and from visceral organ including pancreas. Nociceptive fibres transmitting pain also travel through the celiac plexus. Endoscopic ultrasound allows direct visualization of the celiac plexus region and can even localise the celiac ganglion (Castillo-Roth & Gress, 2010). This enables celiac plexus block to be performed successfully and safely as a non-pharmacological means for pain relief (Avula & Sherman, 2010).

A linear endoendoscope is used to localise the celiac plexus. It's usually found by passing the endoscope to the posterior lesser curve of gastric fundus and tracing down the aorta to locate the celiac artery take-off at about 40 to 50cm from incisors. Doppler mode can be utilised during the block to ensure the absence of vessels in the path of needle insertion

(Castillo-Roth & Gress, 2010). A 22-gauge or 19-gauge EUS fine needle aspiration needle is passed through the biopsy channel towards the celiac axis until the tips is inserted to the level of the celiac trunk. After removing the stylet of the needle, a 10ml syringe is attached to the needle system. Aspiration is then applied to ensure the needle is not inside a blood vessel. Bupivicaine and then triamcinolone are then injected in the celiac space after safe needle position is confirmed (Avula & Sherman, 2010). The agent for celiac plexus block can be injected either bilaterally on both sides of the celiac artery origin or just anterior to the take-off of celiac artery and allow the solution to spread to both sides of the vessels (Castillo-Roth & Gress, 2010). It was shown in randomised controlled trial that there was no difference in the technical success, symptom relief and complication rate between bilateral or single site injections (Leblanc et al., 2009). With the advance in endosonographic imaging, localisation of the celiac ganglia and direct ganglia block is possible. While initial data suggested that this approach was safe and effective in initial pain control (Levy et al., 2008), more studies were awaited to evaluate its long-term efficacy and the optimal drugs to be delivered as compared to conventional percutaneous celiac plexus block.

Concerning the overall efficacy in pain control by EUS-guided celiac plexus block, a metaanlysis showed that approximately 60% of patients reported pain relief after the procedure (Pauli et al., 2009). The exact intensity of pain relief and duration of pain control, however, were not described in the metaanalysis. In a series of 90 patients (Gress et al., 2001) receiving EUS-guided celiac plexus block, only 10% of patients had sustained pain reduction at 6 months. This result suggested that further studies on optimal drugs and treatment regimen would be necessary to improve the success rate. In case of refractory pain despite reinterventions, referral to surgery should be considered.

4. Efficacy of endoscopic treatment

Owing to the variety of endoscopic therapy available and the heterogenous nature of the underlying chronic pancreatitis, outcome of endoscopic treatment has to be considered judiciously. In a retrospective review of 125 patients with 324 intraductal stones (Farnbacher et al., 2002), the technical success rate, as defined by stone fragmentations, was reported to be 85%. However, many of these patients required repeated endoscopic intervention plus ESWL. The complete duct clearance rate was only 51%, whereas, 34% patient had partial clearance. For clinical success rate, defined as pain free after treatment, 52% of patients developed relapses of pain and were hospitalized again for treatment. The causes of recurrent pain were mostly due to recurrent stones or malfunction of the pancreatic stents inserted. Thirteen percent of patients in the series required subsequent surgery due to intractable pain after unsuccessful endoscopic treatment.

There were two randomised controlled trials comparing endoscopic treatment to surgical treatment in patients with chronic pancreatitis and pancreatic ductal stones (Dite et al., 2003; Cahen et al., 2007). Both studies concluded that surgery was superior to endoscopic treatment in achieving long term pain control, but they still recommended the use of endoscopic treatment in some selected cases of chronic pancreatitis with less severe ductal obstruction. The techniques employed in the endoscopic treatment arm in these 2 studies had been criticised. The endoscopic arm in study by Dite et al. did not received ESWL, whereas the endoscopic arm in study by Cahen et al. used stents without side-holes. The latter study was also criticised by the small sample size of total 39 patients (Deviere et al., 2008). Because of the limitation in the randomised controlled studies, endoscopic treatment still played an important role in the management chronic pancreatitis, especially in patients unfit for surgery or refusing surgery (Frulloni et al., 2010). Endoscopic treatment can be proposed as first-line treatment for the following reasons (Khanna & Tandon, 2008) - firstly, it is less invasive than surgery; secondly, it can be repeated in case of relapse of pain; and thirdly, surgery can still be performed in refractory disease as a salvage manoeuvre.

5. Conclusion

Endoscopic therapy can be employed to alleviate pain in patient with chronic pancreatitis. Different endoscopic techniques, including sphincterotomy, stenting, stricture dilatation, stone removal and the insertion of nasopancreatic drain combined with extracorporal shock wave lithotripsy had been described with successful results. The use of endoscopic ultrasound-guided drainage of pseudocyst and celiac plexus block were also important alternative to surgical treatment. With the advance of endoscopic equipment, improvement of techniques and a better understanding of the pathophysiology of chronic pancreatitis, endoscopic treatment might provide patients a less invasive and comparably effective choice of therapy. However, not all patients were rendered sustained symptomatic relief. Patients with persistent pain or pancreatic mass suspicious of malignancy should be referred for consideration of surgical treatment.

6. References

Aghdassi A, Mayerle J, Kraft M, Sielenkämper AW, Heidecke CD, Lerch MM. (2008) Diagnosis and treatment of pancreatic pseudocysts in chronic pancreatitis. *Pancreas,* Vol. 36, No.2, (March 2008), pp. 105-112, ISSN 0885-3177

Avula H & Sherman S. (2010) What is the role of endotherapy in chronic pancreatitis? *Therapeutic Advances in Gastroenterology,* Vol. 3, No. 6, (November 2010), pp. 367-382, ISSN 1756-283X

Baillie J. (2004) Pancreaitic pseudocysts (Part II) *Gastrointestinal Endoscopy,* Vol 60, No. 1, (July 2004), pp. 105-113, ISSN 0016-5107

Binmoeller KF, Seifert H, Walter A, Soehendra N. (1995) Transpapillary and transmural drainage of pancreatic pseudocysts. Gastrointestinal Endoscopy, Vol. 42, No. 3, (September 1995), pp. 219-224, ISSN 0016-5107

Buscaglia JM & Kalloo AN. (2007) Pancreatic sphincterotomy: Technique, indications, and complications. *World Journal of Gasgtroenterology,* Vol.13, No.30, (August 2007), pp. 4064-71, ISSN 1007-9327

Cahen DL, Gouma DJ, Nio Y, Rauws EA, Boermeester MA, Busch OR, Stocker J, Lameris JS, Dijkgraaf MG, Huibregtse K & Bruno MJ. (2007) Endoscopic versus surgical drainage of the pancreatic duct in chronic pancreatitis. *New*

Endland Journal of Medicine, Vol. 356, No. 7, (February 2007), pp. 676-684, ISSN 0028-4793

Castillo-Roth A & Gress F. (2010) Endoscopic ultrasound-guided celiac plexus block and celiac plexus neurolysis, In: *Endoscopic Ultrasound*, Shami VM & Kahaleh M, pp. 425-440, Humana Press, ISBN 978-1-0327-479-1, New York, USA

Cheung YS, Lee KF, Wong J, Ng WW, Chan MF, Chan CK & Lai PB. (2008) Pseudocystectomy: an unusual operation for an atypical pancreatic pseudocyst, *Surgical Practice*, Vol. 12, No. 1, (February 2008), pp. 30-33, ISSN 1744-1633

Costamagna G, Gabbrielli A, Mutignani M, Perri Vincenzo, Pandolfi M, Boscaini M & Crucitti F. (1997) Extracorporeal shock wave lithotripsy of pancreatic stones in chronic pancreiatitis: immediate and medium-term results. *Gastrointestinal Endoscopy*, Vol. 46, No.3, (September 1997), pp. 231-236, ISSN 0016-5107

Choi KS & Kim MH. (2006) Extracorporeal shock wave lithotripsy for the treatment of pancreatic ductal stones. *Journal of Hepato-Biliary-Pancreatic Surgery*. Vol. 13, No. 2, (April 2006), pp. 86-93, ISSN 1868-6974

Dite P, Ruzicka M, Zboril V & Novotny I. (2003) A prospective, randomized trial comparing endoscopic and surgical therapy for chronic pancraitits. *Endoscopy*, Vol. 35, No. 7, (July 2003), pp553-558, ISSN 0013-726X

Farnbacher M, Schoen C, Rabenstein T, Benninger J, Hahn E & Schneider T. (2002) Pancreatic duct stones in chronic pancreatitis: criteria for treatment intensity and success. *Gastrointestinal Endoscopy*, Vol. 56, No. 4, (October 2002), pp. 501-506, ISSN 0016-5107

Frulloni L, Falconi M, Gabbrielli A, Gaia E, Graziani R, Pezzilli R, Uomo G, Andriulli, Balzano G, Benini L, Calculli L, Campra D, Capurso G, Cavestro GM, Angelis CD, Ghezzo L, Manfredi R, Malesci A, ariani A, Mutignani M, Vntrucci , Zamboni G, Amodia A & Vantini I. (2010) Italian consensus guidelines for chroni pancreatitis. *Digestive and Liver Disease*, Vol. 42 Suppl. 6, (November 2010), pp. S381-S406. ISSN 1590-8658

Gress F, Schmitt C, Sherman S, Ciaccia D, Ikenberry S, Lehman G. (2001) Endoscopic ultrasound-guided celiac plexus block for managing abdominal pain associated with chronic pancreatitis: a prospective single center experience. The American Journal of Gastroenterology, Vol. 96, No. 2, (2001), pp. 409 – 416, ISSN 0002-9270

Hirai T, Goto H, Hirooka Y, Itoh A, Hashimoto S, Niwa Y & Hayakawat. (2004) Pilot study of pancreatoscopic lithotripsy using a 5-Fr instrument: selected patients may benefit. *Endoscopy*, Vol. 36, No. 3, (March 2004), pp. 212-216, ISSN 0013-726X

Howell DA, Dy RM, Hanson BL, Nezhad SF & Broaddus SB. (1999) Endoscopic treatment of pancreatic duct stones using a 10F pancreatoscope and electrophydraulic lithotripsy. *Gastrointestinal Endoscopy*, Vol. 50, No. 6, (December 1999), pp.829-833, ISSN 0016-5107

Itoi T, Itokawa F, Tsuchiya T, Kawai T & Moriyasu F. (2009) EUS-guided pancreatic pseudocyst drainage: simultaneous placement of stents and nasocystic catheter using double-guidewire technique. *Digestive Endoscopy*, Vol. 21, Suppl. 1, (July 2009),pp. S53-S56. ISSN 1443-1661

Khanna S & Tandon RK. (2008) Endotherapy for pain in chronic pancreatitis. *Journal of Gastroenterology and Hepatology*, Vol. 23, No.11, (November 2008), pp1649-1656. ISSN 1440-1746

Lai PB, Leung KN, Chan AC, Leok CK & Lau WY. (1997) Case 18. Rupture of a splenic artery pseudoaneurysm into a pancreatic pseudocyst. *Canadian Journal of Surgery*, Vol. 40, No.6, (December 1997), pp. 412, 430. ISSN 0008-428X

Lawrence C, Siddiqi MF, Hamilton JN, Keane TE, Romagnulol J, Hawes RH & Cotton P.B. (2010) Chronic Calcific Pancreatitis: Combination ERCP and Extracorporeal Shock Wave litotripsy for pancreatic ductal stones. *Southern Medical Jounrnal*, Vol. 13, No. 6, (June 2010), pp.505-508, ISSN 0038-4348

LeBlanc JK, DeWitt J, Johnson C, Okumu W, McGreevy K, Symms M, McHenry L, Sherman S & Imperiale T. (2009) A prospective randomized trial of 1 versus 2 injections furing EUS-guided celiac plexus block for chronic pancreaitits pain. *Gastrointestestinal Endoscopy*, Vol. 69, No. 4, (April 2009), pp. 835-842, ISSN 0016-5107

Levy MJ, Topanzian MD, Wiersema MJ, Clain JE, Rajan E, Wang KK, de la Mora JG, Gleeson FC, Pearson RK, Pelaez Mc, Petersen BT, Vege SS & Chari ST. (2008) Initial evaluation of the efficacy and safety of endoscopic ultrasound-guided direct ganglia neurolysis and block. *American Journal of Gastroenterology*, Vol.103 No. 1 , (January 2008), pp. 98-103, ISSN 0002-9270

Puli SR, Reddy JB, Bechtold ML, Antillon MR & Brugge WR. (2009) EUS-guided celiac plexus neurolysis for pain due to chronic pancreatitis or pancreatic cancer pain: a meta-analysis and systematic review. *Digestive Diseases and Sciences*, Vol. 54, No.11, (November 2009), pp.2330-2337, ISSN 0163-2116

Schnelldorfer T, Lewin DN & Adams DB. (2007) Operative management of chronic pancreaitits: longterm results in 372 patients. *Journal of American College of Surgeons*, Vol. 204, No.5, (May 2007), pp. 1039-1047, ISSN 1072-7515

Seewald S, Ang TL, Tend KC & Soehendra N. (2009) EUS-guided drainage of pancreatic pseudocysts, abscesses and infected necrosis. *Digestive Endoscopy*, Vol. 21, Suppl. 1, (July 2009), pp S61-S65, ISSN 1443-1661

Sherman S & Lehman GA (1998). Endoscopic treatment of chronic pancreatitis, In: *Surgical diseases of the pancreas 3rd Ed*, Howard J, Idezuki Y, Ihse I & Prinz R, (Ed.), pp. 343-357, Williams & Silkins, ISBN 0683180193, Maryland, USA.

Strobel O, Buchler MW & Werner J. (2009) Surgical therapy of chronic pancreaittiis: Indications, techniques and results. *International journal of Surgery*, Vol. 7, No. 4, (August 2009), pp. 305-312, ISSN 1743-9191

Tarnasky PR, Hoffman B, Aabakken L, Knapple WL, Coyle W, Pineau B, Cunningham JT, Cotton PB, Hawes RH. (1997) Sphincter of Oddi dysfunction is associated with chronic pancreatitis. The American Journal of Gastroenterology, Vol. 92, No.7, (July 1997), pp. 1125-1129, ISSN 0002-9270

Yoo BM & Lehman GA. (2009) Update on endoscopic treatment of chronic pancreatitis. *Korean Journal of Internal Medicine*, Vol. 24, No. 3, (September 2009), pp. 169-179, ISSN 1226-3303

6

Surgical Options for Chronic Pancreatitis

Fazl Q. Parray[1], Mehmood A. Wani[2] and Nazir A. Wani[3]
[1]*Additional Professor,*
[2]*Post doctoral student Lakesure tertiary care Hospital Kochi India*
[3]*Ex Dean Faculty and Chairman Surgical Division*
Department of Surgery, Sheri-Kashmir Institute of Medical Sciences, India

1. Introduction

The early teaching used to be "Eat when you can, sleep when you can and don't operate on the pancreas". Also the belief was that God put the pancreas at the back because He did not want surgeons messing with it. It was Rufus of Ephesus (c. 100AD) who named the organ "Pancreas" (in Greek Pan: all, Kreas: Flesh or meat). Then it was Homer who used the word 'sweetbread" broadly to describe animal flesh (Modilin IM *et al.* Int Hepato-pancreato-biliary association, Indian Chapter, single theme conference; 2002; 1-3:32-46). This organ with the name sweetbread, however, turns quite bitter as soon it develops the pathological condition called chronic pancreatitis. H. Durmen has summarized the anatomical relationship of the pancreas as: "The pancreas cuddles the left kidney, tickles the spleen, hugs the duodenum, cradles the aorta, opposes the inferior vena cava, dallies with the right renal pedicle, hides behind the posterior parietal peritoneum of the lesser sac and wraps itself around the superior mesenteric vessels"(Dionigi R *et al*). It derives its blood supply from major branches of the celiac and superior mesenteric arteries and it is mandatory for any surgeon operating on the pancreas to develop understanding of its vascular anatomy and its possible variations.

Chronic pancreatitis has been defined as a continuing inflammatory disease of the pancreas characterized by irreversible morphologic changes that typically cause pain and or permanent loss of function (Clain JE, Pearson RK. Surg Clinc North Am 1999;79:829-46). An ideal classification system for chronic pancreatitis would be simple, objective, accurate, incorporating etiology, pathogenesis, structure, function and clinical status into one overall scheme. Although these criteria have never been met, several systems have been advocated. The most widely used classification systems include Marseille classification of 1963 (Sarles H.Symposium of Marseille 1963. Besel),with revisions in 1984 and 1987 and the Cambridge classification of 1984 (Sarner M and Cotton PB. Gut 1984;24:756-9). The Cambridge system proves more useful as a staging system once the diagnosis has been established. The Marseille-Rome classification 1987 includes more causal factors but proves to be more useful in defining pancreatitis. The numbers have increased markedly probably due to the changes in alcohol consumption and improved sensitivity of diagnostic tests. Early series from Copenhagen (Copenhagen pancreatitis study. Scand J Gastroenterol 1981;16:305-12), the

U.S.(Reila A *et al.* Mayo clin Proc 1992;67:839-45) and Mexico City(Robles-Diaz G *et al;* Pancreas 1990;5:479-83) reported a similar incidence of about 4 per 100,000 inhabitants per year and prevalence rate of 45.5 per 100,000 in males and 12.4 per 100,000 in females (Charles S T, Singer MV. Scand J Gastrenterol 2003; 35:136-41). Recent advances in techniques and genetics provide possibilities for early and accurate identification of risk factors leading to chronic pancreatitis. Chronic pancreatitis has been categorized into toxic, idiopathic, genetic, autoimmune, recurrent attacks of acute pancreatitis and obstructive (TIGAR-O risk factor classification system version 1). The classification is based on prevalence of each etiological factor and has implications for potential treatment.

2. Pathogenesis

The hallmark of chronic pancreatitis is the replacement of normal pancreatic tissue with fibrotic tissue. This change leads to mass formation, ductal obstruction, and encasement of other structures or some combination of the above (Amman RW *et al.* Gastroenterology 1984; 86:820-8).The mechanism by which fibrosis takes place is incompletely understood but several advances have been made in the last several years. Ethanol in alcohol or its metabolites are believed to have a direct toxic effect on the pancreas and contribute to the development of chronic pancreatitis (Levy P *et al.* Pancreas 1995; 10:231-8). Ethanol seems to stimulate Pancreatic stellate cells (PSCs) through its metabolite acetaldehyde. PSCs regulate extracellular matrix proteins within the pancreas and collagen deposition within the gland. PSCs also in response to and production of various cytokines results in a self-sustaining cycle of inflammation and fibrosis (Apte MV,Wilson JS. Pancreas 2003; 27:316-20). Pancretic stone protein (PSP), or lithostathine, is also effected by ethanol and may be over or underproduced in patients of chronic pancreatitis.The role of PSP is to stabilize inorganic ion complexes and to prevent precipitation of calcium carbonate (Bernard JP *et al.* Gastroenterology 1992; 103:1277-84). Alterations in PSP productions can lead to protein plugs or pancreatic duct stones which in turn can lead to ductal obstruction, intraductal and parenchymal hypertension, and subsequent continued cellular and organ damage. Many people over- consume ethanol and still do not develop the disease in contrary to those who consume very little and still develop the disease. The most likely explanation for this is that some patients are born with or develop a genetic predisposition and get the disease by a multistep complex pathway. Several genetic aberrancies have been well implicated like PRSS1, SPINK1, and CFTR and are considered to be most notable for the development of chronic pancreatitis.PRSS1 is involved in trypsin metabolism and regulation of the conversion of pro-pancreatic enzymes to their active form. SPINK1 inhibits intrapancreatic trypsin function to help autodigestion. The cystic fibrosis transcription repair (CFTR) gene is an essential gene for the proper regulation of pancreatic fluid, calcium and bicarbonate secretion. Regulation of bicarbonate also effects the inactive versus active forms of trypsin. The net effect of all these processes is chronic injury to the parenchyma of the pancreas with subsequent fibrosis and collagen deposition. Although this accounts, at least in part, for the mass effect in some patients and for the intraductal and glandular hypertension but may not completely explain why some patients have pain syndromes and others do not. The pathogenesis of pain is almost certainly linked in some degree to the already mentioned facts but still some patients have the disease without any mass effect or any evidence of ductal obstruction (Martin RF and Marion MD. Surg Clinic N Am 2007; 87:1461-1475).

Medical management which consists of enzyme replacement, control of diabetes with insulin and oral analgesics is generally effective, although eventually one third of the patients will need surgery during the course of their disease. The surgical management of pancreatitis has seen its ups and downs over the past few decades.

The risks of pancreatic surgery were initially high but a few surgeons were bold enough to approach the chronically inflamed and enlarged pancreas. A number of surgical procedures have been developed during the 20th century to deal with the condition. Review of literature indicates the maximum efficacy of any procedure to be 85 to 90%. There is no procedure evolved to provide a 100% cure for the condition. (Udani PM *et al* <http/bhjorg/journal/1999:4102>)

Dr. Kenneth Warren reported in 1959 that operations for chronic pancreatitis failed when they were not chosen on the basis of pathology observed at the time of operation and all operations were not successful all the time. His statements hold true even for present time (Warren KW. Gastroenterology 1959; 36:224-31). Therefore, surgery is aimed at controlling pain and managing complications rather than halting the progression of the disease. An appropriate and effective procedure has been difficult to devise and at the moment there is no clear "market leader" operation and the choice depends up on a grey zone where in pathological picture, patient's condition and available expertise dictate the final procedure the patient undergoes. The trends in choice of operation have not solely been based on better capacity to match the operation with the pathology discovered in the patient but also with the global level of comfort with the operations being performed. The ideal procedure for treating pain in chronic pancreatitis should be the one which is simple, easy to perform, associated with low morbidity and mortality, and at the same time should provide adequate drainage and not augment endocrine and exocrine insufficiency.

3. Indications for surgical intervention

Currently the following are considered the acceptable indications for surgery (Knoeful WT *et al*. Panceratology 2002; 2:379-85).

1. Intractable pain.
2. Suspicion of malignant neoplasm.
3. Non-resolving ductal stenosis.
4. Non-resolving common bile duct stenosis.
5. Pseudo-aneurysms or vascular erosions not controlled by radiological intervention.
6. Endoscopically not controlled large pseudopancreatic cyst.
7. Intractable internal pancreatic fistula.

4. Preoperative evaluation and patient selection

Once a patient has been selected to undergo surgery for pain relief, a thorough preoperative evaluation must be performed. Two important questions must be answered.

1. Will this patient benefit most from a decompression of the pancreatic ductal system or from resection of pancreas?
2. Is this patient harboring a pancreatic malignancy?

The various biochemical and radiological tests for preoperative assessment and diagnosis are as follows.

4.1 Blood tests

Elevations of serum amylase and lipase are found helpful during acute attacks of pain. In the later stages chronic pancreatitis atrophy of the pancreatic parenchyma can result in serum enzyme levels within the reference range, even during acute exacerbations.

While low levels of serum trypsin are specific for advanced chronic pancreatitis, they are not sensitive enough to be helpful in most patients with mild to moderate disease.(Yashke P-e medicine)

Laboratory studies to identify causative factors include serum calcium and triglyceride levels.

4.2 Fecal tests

Steatorrhoea may be present in advanced chronic pancreatitis but neither qualitative nor quantitative fecal fat analysis can detect early disease.

4.3 Direct tests

Tests to detect chronic pancreatitis early are invasive and expensive.

4.3.1 Determination of duodenal aspirates

Pancreatic secretions are stimulated by exogenous secretion to achieve maximal output. The bicarbonate, protease, amylase and lipase output is then measured in the duodenal aspirates. This test is, however, only available in specialized centers.

4.3.2 Determination in pancreatic juice

This test is performed at the time of endoscopic retrograde pancreatography (ERCP). The pancreatic duct is freely cannulated, an external secretagogue is administered and the pancreatic juice is then aspirated out of the duct as it is produced. The bicarbonate, protease, amylase and lipase output is then measured. This test is gaining popularity because most patients undergo ERCP during the evaluation of chronic pancreatitis.

4.4 Indirect test

Non-invasive tests in principle work via oral administration of a complex substance that is hydrolyzed by a specific pancreatic enzyme to release a marker substance. The marker is then absorbed by the intestine and in turn measured in the serum or urine. These tests are capable of detecting moderate to severe degrees of chronic pancreatitis. Liver, renal and intestinal disease may interfere with the interpretation of these tests. They are not freely available in the United States (Yashke P e-medicine; Laukoisch PG. Int J Pancreatol 1993 Aug; 14(1):9-20).

4.5 Imaging studies

Structural changes in the pancreas and its ductal system are only seen during the moderate and severe stages of the disease, so most imaging procedures cannot depict early chronic pancreatitis.

4.5.1 Abdominal radiograph

Pancreatic calcification is observed in 30% of cases. They first form in the head and then in body and tail. Paired anterposterior and oblique views are preferred because the vertebral column may otherwise obscure small specks of calcification.

4.5.2 Computerized tomography

Although CT excels at depicting the morphological changes of advanced chronic pancreatitis, the early changes are beyond its resolution and a normal finding on this study does not rule out chronic pancreatitis. CT is most useful to identify complications and in planning surgical or endoscopic intervention (Yashke P, e-medicine).

4.5.3 Endoscopic retrograde pancreatography (ERCP)

ERCP provides the most accurate visualization of the pancreatic ductal system and has been regarded as the criterion standard for diagnosing chronic pancreatitis. Conversely one limitation of ERCP is that it cannot be used to evaluate the pancreatic parenchyma, and histologically proven chronic pancreatitis has been documented in the setting of normal pancreatogram. The pancreatogram can be classified according to several schemes such as Cambridge criteria (Laukisch etal.Pancreas 1996 Mar;12(2):149-52).

A comparison of pancreatogram scoring with direct pancreatic function tests demonstrates good correlation. However, pancreatography tended to show more significant severe changes. ERCP is invasive, expensive, requires complete opacification of the pancreatic duct to visualize side branches and carries a risk of pancreatitis (Yashke P, e-medicine; Catalano MF *et al.* Gastrointestinal Endoscop 1998 Jul;48(1):11-7(medline).

4.5.4 Magnetic resonance cholangiopancreatography (MRCP)

MRCP imaging provides information on the pancreatic parenchyma and adjacent abdominal viscera and uses heavily T2 weighted images to visualize the biliary and pancreatic ductal system. The use of secretin during the procedure enhances the quality to enable the diagnosis of early chronic pancreatitis; however, it is relatively safe, reasonably accurate, non-invasive, fast and very useful in planning surgical and endoscopic intervention (Yashke P, e-medicine; Sota JA *et al.* AJR Am J Roentgenol 1995;165(6):1397-401(medline).

4.5.5 Endoscopic ultrasound (EUS)

EUS may be the best test for imaging the pancreas as per the recent studies. By placing the transducer immediately adjacent to the pancreas, the endoscopic approach eliminates the interference by bowel gas and enables the use of high frequency probes to enable acquisition of detailed imaging. Eleven sonographic criteria have been developed that identify characteristic findings of chronic pancreatitis. Using these criteria EUS correlates well with endoscopic pancreatic ductography and intra-ductal secretin tests in moderate and severe disease. EUS may be useful in diagnosing chronic pancreatitis in a subset of patient with non-ulcer dyspepsia. More experience is required to determine its utility in detecting the early stages of chronic pancreatitis (Yashke P, e-medicine; Catalano MF *et al.* Gastrointestinal Endoscop 1998 Jul;48(1):11-7(medline). The new Rosemont criteria, using a combination of major and/or minor criteria, categorizes the patient as having EUS features that are (1) consistent with chronic pancreatitis, (2) suggestive of chronic pancreatitis, (3) indeterminate of chronic pancreatitis, (4) normal.

The researchers concluded that the new Rosemont classification system represents an improvement over current means of EUS diagnosis for chronic pancreatitis. They acknowledge the results of their deliberations do not provide a validation of their recommendations, but intend to apply these criteria in a manner that provides easy and reproducible means of EUS diagnosis and grading of chronic pancreatitis so that they may be used to help guide patient care and future study design. In an accompanying editorial, Walter G. Park, MD, and ASGE President Jacques Van Dam, MD, PhD, FASGE, division of gastroenterology, Stanford University Medical Center, Cal., state that "despite being less than the perfect criterion standard, it remains the best to date"(EUS-Based Criteria For The Diagnosis Of Chronic Pancreatitis: The Rosemont Classification,*ScienceDaily (June 29, 2009)* American Society for Gastrointestinal Endoscopy).

4.6 Other tests

A secretin stimulated ultrasound study is one way of looking for the resistance to pancreatic juice outflow at the level of the duodenum. The diameter of the pancreatic duct is measured at baseline and then 15 and 30 min after injection of secretin. Dilatation to a diameter greater than normal or for a longer period implies the presence of periampullary stricture or papillary stenosis (Yashke P,e-medicine; Catalano MF *et al.* Gastrointestinal Endoscop 1998 Jul;48(1):11-7(medline).

5. What is the most appropriate procedure?

The choice of surgical procedure depends upon the indication for surgery and the characteristics of disease in the individual patient. In general it is most appropriate to select a procedure which is likely to achieve the maximum symptomatic pain relief and also maximally preserve the functional pancreatic tissue.(Wani NA *et al.* Int J Surg 2007;5:45-56).

Drainage procedures were developed on the basis that the pain in chronic pancreatitis is due to ductal hypertension (Ebbehoj N *et al.*Scand J Gastroenterol 1984;19:1066-8) and proper drainage could decompress it. On the other hand the theories of perineural inflammation as the cause of pain lead to the development of resectional procedures (Bockmann DE. Gastroenterology 1988;94;1459-69).

5.1 Drainage procedure

1. **Partial**: draining the duct partially,
    a. Sphincterotomy and sphincteroplasty,
    b. Duval procedure,
    c. Puestow Gillesby procedure,
    d. Leger's procedure,
    e. Marcadier procedure,
2. **Complete**: draining the main duct completely,
    I. Pancreaticojejunostomy,
        a. PartingtonRochelle procedure,
        b. Bapat's modification of Partington's procedure,
    II. Pancreaticogastrostomy,
        a. Moreno Gonzales procedure.

5.2 Resectional procedures

a. Whipple's operation,
b. Traversoe Longmire procedure,
c. Begar's procedure,
d. Berne modification,
e. Denervated pancreatic flap,
   Warrens denervated pancreatic flap,
   Shires denervated splenopancreatic flap,
f. Subtotal pancreatic resection,
g. Childs procedure,
h. Total pancreatectomy,
   With duodenal preservation,
   Without duodenal preservation.

5.3 Extended drainage procedure

a. Rumpf's extended drainage.

5.4 Resection with extended drainage

a. Extended Begar's procedure,
b. Frey's procedure,
c. Izbicki V shaped ventral pancreatic excision.

5.5 Pancreatic denervation alone

a. Left splanchnicectomy with celiac ganglionectomy,
b. Left splanchnicectomy, celiac ganglionectomy with bilateral vagotomy,
c. Complete pancreatic denervation,
d. Transthoracic / videothoracoscopic pancreatic denervation:

5.6 Pancreatic auto-transplantation

a. Islet cell transplantation,
b. Segmental pancreatic transplantation.

Drainage procedures

These drainage procedures gave pain relief in up to 60-80% cases (Udani PM *et al*<http/bhjorg/journal /1999: 4102>).

Partial drainage procedures

Sphincterotomy and sphincteroplasty

Transduodenal sphincterotomy was originally proposed by Doubilet and Mulholland for the treatmentof chronic pancreatitis with the mistaken belief that the disease was caused by bile reflux (Doubilet H *et al.* J Am Med Assoc 1956;160:521-8).The operation did not prove effective and subsequent attempts to improve pancreatic drainage by dividing the septum between the bile duct and the pancreatic duct have not proved popular (Bartlet MK *et al.*New Engl J Med 1960;262:642-8). In chronic pancreatitis it is unusual to find a uniformly dilated duct obstructed at the termination only therefore it follows that these procedures are unlikely to prove successful; however, early success rates of 50% (Doubilet H *et al.* J Am Med Assoc 1956;160:521-8 Bartlet MK *et al.* New Engl J Med 1960;262:642-8) when pain relief was assessed at 5 years have not been sustained (Bagley FH *et al.*Am J Surg 1981;141:418-21) Although surgical sphincterotomy has largely been given up; similar procedures have been performed endoscopically in the past with enthusiasm (Grim H *et al.*Endoscopy 1989;21:70-4).

Duval procedure

Decompression of the main pancreatic duct is achieved by resection of the pancreatic tail and retrograde drainage of the pancreatic duct via a termino-lateral pancreaticojejunostomy (Figure 1).

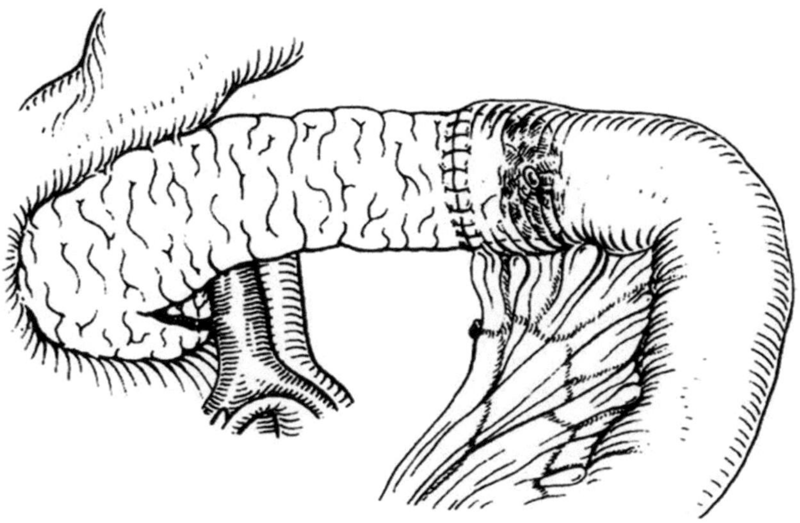

Fig. 1. Duval Procedure

However, this procedure will only be effective if there is a single stricture between pancreatic tail and the ampulla of Vater which in most of the cases is unlikely (Duval MK. Ann Surg 1954;140:775-85).

Puestow Gillesby procedure

They recommend a longitudinal opening of the pancreatic duct from the site of the transaction of the duct after resection of the pancreatic tail and spleen to a point to the right of the mesenteric vessels and invagination of the open duct with pancreas into a Roux-en-Y loop of jejunum, thus ensuring a wider drainage of the ductal system. This procedure takes care of multiple strictures seen in chronic pancreatitis (Puestow CB *et al.* Arch Surg 1958;76:898-906).

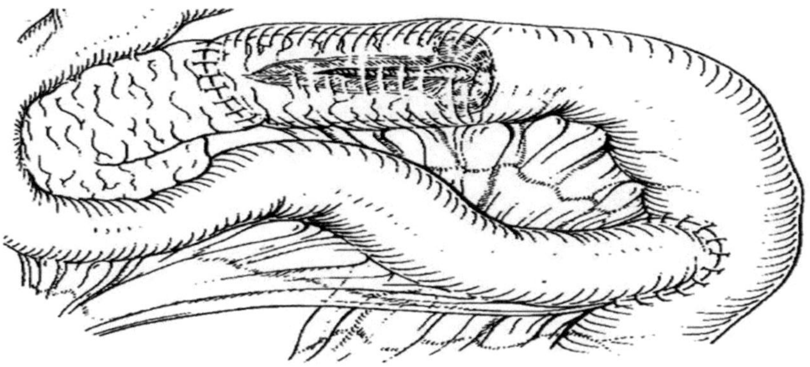

Fig. 2. Puestow Gillsby Procedure

Leger's procedure

This procedure developed for distal strictures involves a 40% distal pancreatectomy with splenectomy followed by opening of the pancreatic duct into a loop of jejunum by a retrograde lateral pancreaticojejunostomy (Leger L *et al.* Ann Surg 1974;180:180-91).

Mercadier procedure

Here only the body of the pancreas is drained into a Roux-en-Y loop of jejunum by a side to side anastamosis (Udani PM *et al*<http/bhjorg/journal/1999:4102>).

Partial drainage procedures have been abandoned because of the small anastamosis which tends to occlude. Also the concept of preservation of the spleen with pancreatic tail is important as it prevents post-splenectomy sepsis(Govil S *et al.* Br J Surg 1999;86(7):895-8) and delays the onset of diabetes mellitus (Withigen J *et al.* Ann Surg 1974;179:412-8).

Complete drainage procedures

Pancreaticojejunostomy

Partington Rochelle procedure. This procedure is a refined Puestow procedure. It consists of a side to side long pancreaticojejunostomy, at least 10 cm without, resection of the pancreatic tail or the pancreas. However, a dilated main pancreatic duct (minimum 8 mm) is a prerequisite for a good duct to mucosa anastamosis (Partington RF *et al.* Ann Surg 1960;152:1037-42). In one of the largest series Greenlee (Grenlee HB *et al.* World J Surg

1990;14:70-6) reported significant improvement in 82% of there patients with lateral pancreaticojejunostomy with an extended follow up of up to 25 years. Similar results have been reported by others (Leger L *et al.* Ann Surg 1974;180:180-91;Moreno-Gonzales I *et al.* Br J Surg 1982;69:254). In our experience, this procedure has been performed on more than 130 patients of chronic pancreatitis with a duct size of more than 7 mm since 1985 till date. We strongly are in favour of this procedure in any patient with a duct size of more than 7 mm because of the technical ease, low morbidity, and excellent long-term results. We observed significant long-term improvement in more than 80% of our patients operated at Sher-i-Kashmir Institute of Medical Sciences,Srinagar,Jammu and Kashmir,India.

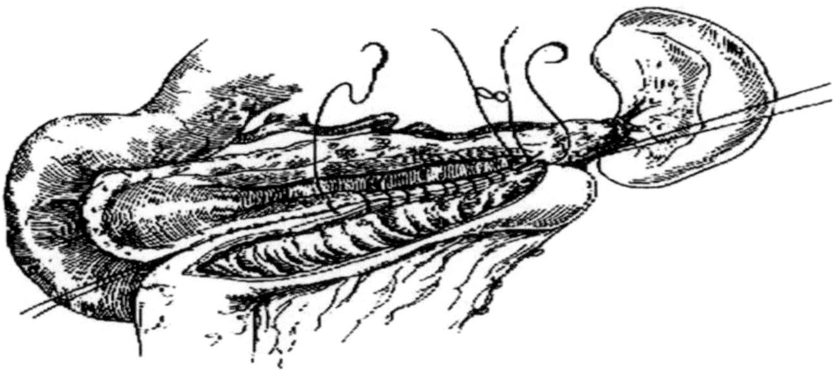

Fig. 3. The Partington Rochelle procedure

Bapat's procedure. It is modification of Partington's procedure. Here the pancreatic duct is opened from head to tail with wide drainage by a side to end pancreaticojejunostomy after fish mouthing the jejunal end to a required length. A duct to mucosa anastamosis is performed. Again the prerequisite is a dilated duct of at least 7 mm. This procedure is more physiological and ensures a straight conical dependent anastamosis with effective and complete drainage (Bapat RD. Indian J Gastroenterol 1997 Jul;16(3):119-20).

Pancreaticogastrostomy

Pancreaticogastrostomy has been advocated by some to be a better form of drainage procedure than pancreaticojejunostomy (Pain JA *et al.* Br J Surg 1988;75:220-22). The procedure is performed as a mucosa to mucosa anastamosis over a T tube. A pain relief of up to 79% has been reported (Jordan GL *et al.* Am J Surg 1977;133:46-50); however, more patients developed steatorrhoea because of the inactivation of the pancreatic enzymes by gastric acid. However,most surgeons still regard pancreaticojejunostomy as the drainage operation of choice.

Moreno Gonzales procedure

Pancreatic and bile duct drainage is established into an isolated vascularised loop of jejunum which is then anastamosed to the duodenum. The procedure has potential advantages, it allows the return of bile and pancreatic secretions into the duodenum and there is no pancreaticocibal asynchrony.

In conclusion the patients with ductal dilatation of more than 7-8 mm, no inflammatory mass or ductal abnormality in the head and uncinate process are the most suitable candidates for lateral pancreaticojejunostomy. The results of pancreaticojejunostomy are difficult to interpret. Many reports have differing indications, different forms of surgery and inadequate follow up. In general however, all forms of drainage procedures tend to worsen over time especially if patients do not abstain from alcohol (Lerut JP *et al.* Ann Surg 1984;1999:432-7).

Resectional procedure

The head is considered to be pacemaker of the disease and its complications. A mass in the pancreatic head is found in 30-60% of the patients with chronic pancreatitis (Buchler M *et al.* Am J Surg 1995;169:65-70). No study has yet conclusively shown pain being only attributable to main duct obstruction and it is difficult to think of a good reason to believe so. The pathogenesis of pain is most likely not only related to ductal and parenchymal hypertension but also to the theory of perineural inflammation (Bockmann DE. Gastroenterology 1988;94:1459-69).

In addition lateral pancreaticojejunostomy never drains the second and third order pancreatic ducts, hence the concept led to the development of resectional procedures.

Whipple's operation (1935)

The procedure although first described by Allen O Whipple in 1912, but published much later for malignant lesions of the head of the pancreas is now also used for benign inflammatory mass in the head with a non-dilated pancreatic duct. The procedure consists of a pancreaticoduodenectomy with reconstruction by a pancreaticojejunostomy/ gastrostomy, gastrojejunostomy and choledochojejunostomy. The intellectual basis for the shift in resection of the distal pancreas to that of pancreatic head was the concept of the "Pain Pacemaker" being located in the head of the pancreas promulgated by Dr. Longmires. This is a complex and technically challenging procedure with higher mortality rates as compared to drainage procedure, however, with good results. This procedure involves excising normal organs much against the principles of surgery for a benign disorder and has given way to more conservative approaches (Augusto JB *et al.* The Pancreas) However, it is the preferred surgical option if there is any suspicion of malignancy, as in such a situation there should be no compromise on the radicality of the procedure.

Traversoe Longmire procedure

Originally used in 1994 for a peri-ampullary tumor by Watson(Watson K. Br J Surg 1944;31:368-73) it was subsequently used by Traversoe Longmire for chronic pancreatitis in 1978 (Traverso and Longmire. Surg Gynecol Obstet 1978;156:581-6). As a gastrectomy is avoided and the pylorus and the proximal duodenum are preserved it achieves a better postoperative nutritional status, minimizes postgastrectomy syndromes as well as the incidence of marginal ulceration. For these reasons it has almost become the form of resection for patients requiring pancreaticoduodenectomy in chronic pancreatitis. Recent reports on pancreaticoduodenectomy for chronic pancreatitis have recorded a low mortality rate of 0-1%, significant pain relief of 80-100% (Traverso LW *et al.* Ann Surg 1997;226:429-38). The incidence of diabetes increased from 17 to 44% in the preoperative period to 26-64% in the postoperative period (Traverso LW *et al.* Ann Surg 1997;226:429-38;Rossi RL *et al.* Arch Surg 1987;122:416-20). However, the onset of diabetes on follow up rather than immediately after the surgery suggests progression of the disease rather than the effect of surgery.The procedure got more established after the results of a randomized trial. Two hundred and fourteen patients were randomized to undergo either a standard or a pylorus-preserving Whipple resection. After exclusion of 84 patients on the basis of intraoperative findings, 130 patients (66 standard Whipple operation and 64 pylorus-preserving resection) were entered into the trial. Of these, 110 patients with proven adenocarcinoma (57 standard Whipple and 53 pylorus-preserving resection) were analysed for long-term survival and quality of life. There was no difference in perioperative morbidity. Long-term survival, quality of life and weight gain were identical after a median follow-up of 63·1 (range 4–93) months. At 6 months, capacity to work was better after the pylorus-preserving procedure (77 *versus* 56 per cent; $P = 0{\cdot}019$).The conclusion was that both procedures are equally effective for the treatment of pancreatic and periampullary cancer. Pylorus-preserving Whipple resection offers some minor advantages in the early postoperative period, but not in the long term. The same principle applies to managing chronic pancreatitis by using either of the procedure (Seiler, CA etal. British Journal of Surgery, May 2005; 92,(5): 547–556).

Hans Begar's procedure

This procedure is indicated in chronic pancreatitis with inflammatory mass in the head with medically intractable pain, obstruction of the common bile duct, duodenal stenosis or portal hypertension due to compression of portal vein by inflammatory mass. It is a duodenum sparing resection of the head of the pancreas thus preserving duodenal physiology and normal intestinal continuity which has significance in terms of postoperative nutritional status, blood sugar control and marginal ulceration. Two major steps are involved:

Resection: The pancreas is transected at the border between the head and the body above the superior mesenteric vein leaving a small disk of the head between the common bile duct and the duodenal wall.

Drainage: The body of the pancreas is drained by an end to end pancreaticojejunostomy and the pancreatic head by a side to side anastamosis to the rim of the resection cavity (Yasuda H *et al.* J Biliary Tract Pancreas 1990;11:967-73). The procedure seems to be safe with perioperative mortality of 0-0.8%. Significant relief of pain has been reported in 86-92% of patients. It is not associated with fresh development of diabetes in the early postoperative period. However, existing diabetes may worsen in 10-13% of the patients (Beger HG *et al.* Ann Surg 1999;230:512-23). Even, late diabetes develops in 21% of the patients due to progression of the disease. DPPHR when compared to PPPD has a superior outcome because of better pain control, weight gain, better glucose tolerance and higher insulin secretion capacity (Buchler M *et al.* Am J Surg 1995;169:65-70).

Berne modification: In comparision to Begar's technique this modification spares the dissection of the pancreatic body from the portal vein. After the resection of pancreatic head, a single cavum results which can be anastamosed end to side with a ROUX-en-Y jejunal loop. If stenosis of the intrapancreatic part of the common bile duct cannot be resolved by decompression and resection of the surrounding pancreatic tissue, or if the intrapancreatic portion of the common bile duct is opened accidentally during pancreatic head resection, the wall of the opened bile duct is fixed with single stitches to the surrounding tissues like an opened door and is included in the same anastamosis (Koninger J *et al.* Surgery 2008;143(4):490-98).

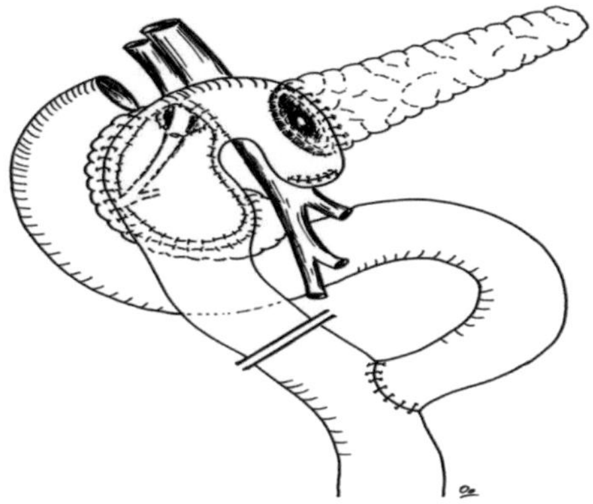

Fig. 4. The Begar's procedure

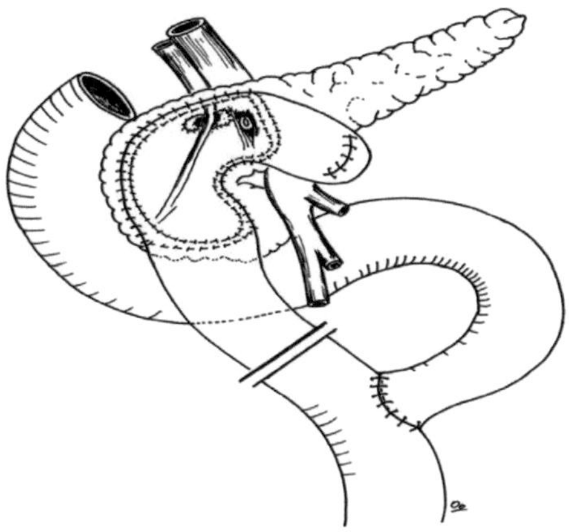

Fig. 5. Berne modification

Denervated pancreatic flaps

In Warrens procedure the pancreas is divided over the portal superior mesenteric vein after ligation of the splenic artery and vein. The pancreatic head is excised leaving a thin rim. The remaining pancreas is not drained. Ligation of splenic vein and artery is presumed to denervate the gland (Warren WD *et al.* Surg Gynecol Obstet 1984;159:581-6). Shires *et al* described a more elaborate procedure called a denervated splenopancreatic flap for patients with small duct pancreatitis (Shires GT *et al.* Ann Surg 1986;203:568). The procedure includes complete mobilization of the pancreas from the retroperitoneum, resection of the head and the uncinate process leaving a small rim near the duodenum, division of the splenic vein near its junction with the superior mesenteric vein and drainage of the distal pancreatic remnant into a Roux-en-Y limb of jejunum. The complexity of the procedure and its unproven efficacy may limit its usefulness.

Subtotal pancreatic resection

Excision of the body and distal pancreas used to be a commonly performed procedure during 1960-1970 but with the development of better imaging facilities it was noted that disease in the body and the tail is often secondary to disease in the head of the pancreas, thereby limiting its role. This procedure is still indicated when the disease is confined to the body and tail e.g., pseudocyst, failed pancreaticojejunostomy, non-dilated duct, pseudo-aneurysm and when there is disease beyond the neck of pancreas, and the pancreatic duct is oversewn. A concomitant splenectomy is unavoidable in the majority of patients because of dense fibrosis precluding the isolation of the splenic vessels. However, splenic preservation may be possible in 20-34% of patients. Another procedure described by Warsaw in which splenic salvage is achieved by preservation of the short gastric vessels; early mortality is 0-4% (Evans TD *et al.* Br J Surg 1997;84:624-9) and pain relief is 70-88% (Frey CF *et al.* Surg Clinc North Am 1989;69:499-528). About 20% develop diabetes in the early postoperative period. Severe hypoglycemic coma and brain damage occur in 2-4% of all such patients (Frey CF *et al.* Surgery of Pancreas 1997;347-55). Further an increased incidence of steatorrhoea is seen in 15% (Frey CF *et al.* Surg Clinc North Am 1989;69:499-528)

Childs resection

This procedure first described by Barret and Bowers in 1957(Barret O *et al.* USAF Med J 1957;8:1037-41); was popularized by Child. It is a 95% distal pancreatectomy. The spleen, the tail, body and uncinate processes are completely removed. The small cuff of the head that is preserved protects the vascularity and common bile duct during surgery. This procedure is performed when lesser procedures have failed or when the entire pancreas is severely diseased (William JF *et al.* Ann Surg 1965;162(4):534-49). Pain relief is about 90% with a mortality of up to 4% while diabetes develops in 50% of patients (Frey CF *et al.* Surgery of Pancreas 1997;347-55) and the incidence of early steatorrhoea increases by 30% (Frey CF *et al.* Surg Clinc North Am 1989;69:499-528).

Total pancreatectomy

Total pancreatectomy bringing in its wake permanent endocrine and exocrine deficiency is usually offered as a last resort to patients with chronic pancreatitis who have diffuse involvement of the pancreas with non-dilated ducts, suspicion of malignancy or failed previous procedure. The operative mortality ranges from 0 to 10% and pain relief is achieved in 80% (Frey CF *et al.* Surg Clinc North Am 1989;69:499-528). In the absence of counter regulatory hormones control of sugar is very difficult (brittle diabetes). Hypoglycemic attacks after total pancreatectomy can lead to death or irreversible brain damage. Patients who are already insulin dependent and need pancreatic supplementation for steatorrhoea are ideally suited for this procedure.

Duodenum preserving total pancreatectomy

Russel in 1987 reported a total pancreatectomy with duodenal preservation. The operative procedure is extremely tedious; pain relief is achieved in 75-80% of patients and no postoperative deaths have been reported. Early complications include bleeding, sepsis and duodenal fistula. However, at a later stage patients may develop bile duct or duodenal stricture. This procedure is also offered as a last report as is total pancreatectomy (Easter DW *et al.* Ann Surg 1991;214:575-80).

Extended drainage procedures

Rumpf's extended drainage procedure

This is a combination of Partington's procedure with a transduodenal pancreatic sphincteroplasty. It is indicated when there is a pre-papillary obstruction to the drainage of pancreatic duct due to stones or stricture (Rumpf KD *et al.* Chirurg 1983;54:722-7).

Resection with extended drainage

The reported incidence of inflammatory mass in the head is about 30% of which only 10% are malignant (Marcus WB *et al.* Am J Surg.1995;169:65-70). Resection with extended drainage procedure provides cure in up to 95% of cases (Izbicki JR *et al.*Ann Surg 1995;221(4):350-8).

Extended Begar's procedure

In cases where there are multiple strictures in the left pancreas with an inflammatory mass in the head, this procedure has a superior result. In addition to the duodenum preserving head resection a side to side pancreaticojejunostomy is performed after slitting open the main pancreatic duct.

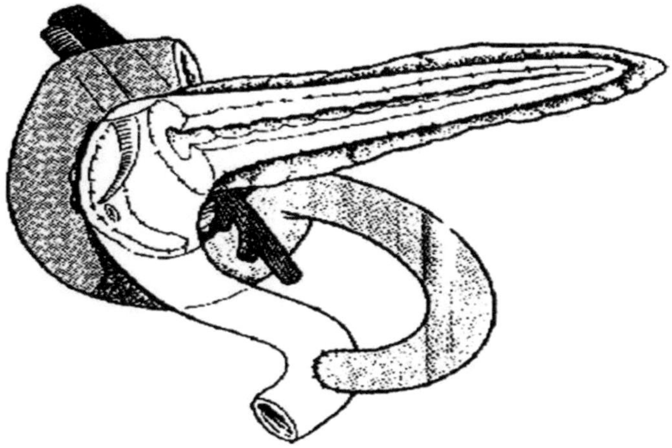

Fig. 6. The Extended Begar's procedure

Frey's procedure

A modified procedure combines lateral pancreaticojejunostomy of Partington Rochelle with coring out of the pancreatic head overlying the ducts of Wirsung and Santorini and the uncinate process using a diathermy, keeping at least 5 mm pancreatic tissue posteriorly and medially. If the duct is less than 8 mm in size mucosa to capsule anastamosis is performed. This procedure is indicated for pain in chronic pancreatitis with its complications like pseudocyst, common bile duct obstruction, pancreatic ascites, fistulae and recurrent pain after lateral pancreaticojejunostomy. It is contraindicated in patients where cancer cannot be excluded (Frey CF. Adv Surg 1999;32:41-85).

Izbicki's "V" shaped ventral pancreatic excision

In this procedure a long "V" shaped excision of ventral aspect of the pancreas is done with a lateral pancreaticojejunostomy by a mucosa to capsule anastamosis. This procedure drains the main as well as the second and third order ducts. This is an ideal procedure for small duct disease with a maximum diameter of the Wirsung's duct less than 3 mm (Izbicki JR *et al.* Ann Surg 1998;227(2):213-14).

Pancreatic denervation alone

Splanchnic nerves and the sympathetic trunks indicate pain arising from the pancreas, extrahepatic biliary ducts and gastrointestinal tract from the level of the stomach to the

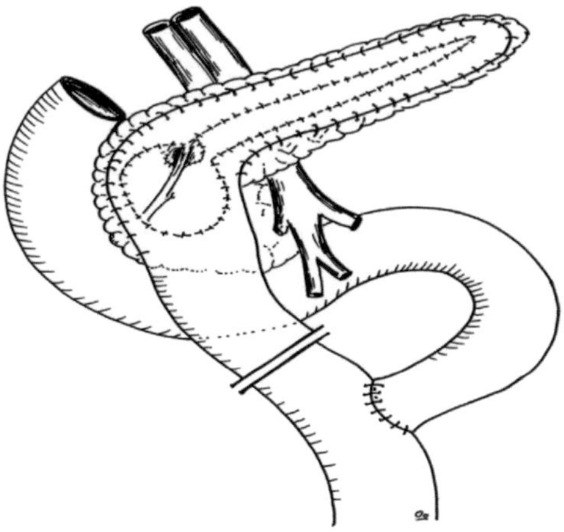

Fig. 7. Duodenum-preserving pancreatic head resection by Frey

rectosigmoid. Interest in surgical neurectomy has progressed by the observation that fibers which mediate pancreatic pain interconnect only through the celiac and superior mesenteric plexus. Various methods of deneravation have been described like left splanchnicectomy with celiac ganglionectomy with or without vagotomy. Mallet Guy advocated an extra peritoneal approach through the 12th rib for left splanchnicectomy with celiac ganglionectomy (Mallet Guy PA. Am J Surg 1983;145:234). This is done after correcting the extra pancreatic pathology. In a 5-year follow up of these patients there was an 84% overall improvement. However, the failure rate was up to 31% in patients with diffuse pancreatic fibrosis and no discernable extra pancreatic cause (White TT *et al.* Am J Surg 1966;112:195). The role of vagal fibers in pancreatic pain is unclear. Generally however, bilateral vagotomy is considered to increase the completeness of pancreatic denervation.

Complete pancreatic denervation

Hirokawa described a more extensive denervation procedure, which includes freeing the pancreas from the posterior abdominal wall and resection of all postganglionic pancreatic nerve plexus including those surrounding the common hepatic and splenic arteries (Hiraoka T *et al.* Am J Surg 1986;152:459). Although there are only a small number of patients who have undergone the procedure and this follow up is short; this procedure may provide a reasonable alternative to extensive resection.

Transthoracic/videothoracoscopic pancreatic denervation

There are important thoracic anatomical considerations regarding the innervation to the pancreas. The greater splanchnic nerves are largely responsible for pain in supramesentric viscera and the nerve trunks lie above the level of the 10th thoracic vertebra and descend along the spine to end in the celiac plexus, similarly the lesser splanchnic plexus. Transthoracic denervation can be achieved by division of the splanchnic nerves with bilateral vagotomy performed through a left thoracotomy. A similar procedure is now performed using a videothoracoscopic technique (Makarewicz W *et al.* World J Surg 2003;27:906-11). This minimally invasive procedure achieved results almost equal to those of major abdominal surgery. Follow up of 12 months demonstrated an improved quality of life. This procedure may be considered for patients who do not meet the anatomic criteria for drainage and those who may not be candidates for major abdominal surgery.

Pancreatic auto-transplantation

Although subtotal and total pancreatectomies successfully alleviate the pain of chronic pancreatitis, patients develop troublesome insulin dependent diabetes mellitus. This can be overcome by auto-transplantation.

Islet cell auto-transplantation

The Mirkowitch technique which is used to prepare partially purified islets produces a fairly large volume of minced digested islet cell tissue which is then injected into a portal vein. Despite slow injection portal pressure is markedly raised several fold. Hinshaw *et al.* developed and tested a more sophisticated islet preparation technique. This technique produced a 5 ml tissue pellet containing 500,000-2000,000 islets for transplantation, no problems were noted with this preparation and the portal pressure remained essentially unchanged. Long-term success (insulin independence) with both these techniques is reported at 40-43% (Hinshaw DB *et al.* Am J Surg 1981;42:118). In recent years total pancreatectomy and islet autotransplantation are done for chronic pancreatitis with intractable pain when other treatment measures have failed, allowing insulin secretory capacity to be preserved, minimizing or preventing diabetes, while at the same time removing the root cause of the pain. Since the first case in 1977, several series have been published. Pain relief is obtained in most patients, and insulin independence preserved long term in about a third, with another third having sufficient beta cell function so that the surgical diabetes is mild. Islet autotransplantation has been done with partial or total pancreatectomy for benign and premalignant conditions. Islet autotransplantation should be used more widely to preserve beta cell mass in major pancreatic resections (Blondet JJ,et al. (2007), *Surgical Clinics of North America,* 87(6): 1477-1501).

Segmental pancreatic transplantation

This technique comprises auto-transplantation of the resected body and tail of the pancreas into the thigh following near total pancreatectomy. The splenic vessels are anastamosed to the femoral vessels. The divided end of the pancreas is closed and the duct is ligated or injected with synthetic polymers (e.g., prolamine or neoprene). Duct obliteration is thought to cause rapid and permanent atrophy of the exocrine pancreas and preserves endocrine function. However, others concluded that duct obliteration does not prevent relapse or progression of chronic pancreatitis in the preserved pancreatic segment. Internal drainage of the duct into a Roux-en-Y limb of jejunum has also been reported with good results. Technical success was achieved in up to 80% of patients with pain relief in 80% and insulin independence in 70% (Rossi RL *et al.* Ann Surg 1986;203:626).

Laparoscopic pancreatic resection

Laparoscopic resection of the pancreas is technically quite demanding and most of the surgeons may find it cumbersome and time consuming, hence their adoption has been limited. Although the operation is technically feasible, the benefit of the laparoscopic approach may not be as apparent as that of a less complex laparoscopic procedure (Gagner M et al. Surg Endosc 1994;8(5):408-10).Recent years have seen an increasing trend in the use of laparoscopy for distal pancreatic resection with splenic preservation. In most studies it has been found that distal pancreas resection can be performed as a laparoscopic procedure, with the usual advantages that this techniques has for the patient. Optimal closure of the cut edge of the pancreas and the preservation of the spleen and its main vessels are the most important aspects of this operation (Uranues S,et al. The American Journal of Surgery, Aug 2006;192(2):257-261). Of late surgeons have started comparing the results of robotic surgery versus laparoscopic surgery in pancreatitis which continues still to be in its infancy because of little evidence at present available in literature (Samuel M,et al ,Pancreas(Oct 2010); 39(7): 1109-1111).

6. Ruling out a malignant neoplasm

There is evidence to suggest that chronic pancreatitis could predispose to pancreatic malignancy (Lowenfels AB *et al.* New England J Med 1993;328:1433-7). Studies show that the risk rises with duration from 1.8% at 10 years to 4% at 20 years and it has been speculated that it is due to the increased levels of growth factors(Kore M *et al.* Gut 1994;35:1468-73); another report showed a 6% malignant change of inflammatory head mass at 9 years follow up (Beger HG *et al.* Ann Surg 1999;230:512-23). Concomitant malignancy has been reported in 15-21% of patients undergoing surgery for chronic pancreatitis which may be detected at surgery or on follow up (Ramesh H. Br J Surg 1992;79:544-9). Differentiating a malignant neoplasm in the head of the pancreas from an inflammatory mass of chronic pancreatitis is a major challenge for the surgeon which needs to be addressed at the time of surgery. The head in chronic pancreatitis is hard and enlarged so the hope of detecting carcinoma by palpation is not possible and is only an illusion. A 15% error in sampling as well as interpretation makes frozen section an unreliable tool to exclude malignancy (Campanale RP *et al.* Arch Surg 1985;12:283-8). Therefore a high degree of suspicion is to be entertained in these patients. In such a situation only resection probably pancreaticoduodenectomy should be preferred as any lesser procedure may leave behind the lesion or cause tumor spillage. Frequently, there bypass procedures become necessary after lateral pancreaticojejunostomy. With pylorus preserving resections these additional procedures are not required. This safely and effectively combines the control of complications with the preservation of original anatomy and thus is a more physiological procedure. The relevance of segmental portal hypertension in a patient of chronic pancreatitis is poorly understood. Complications of segmental portal hypertension are rare and its presence should not influence the choice of operation. Complications such as internal fistula, pseudocysts, pancreatico-portal fistula, or pseudoaneurysm require an individualized approach.

7. Conclusion

In conclusion Chronic pancreatitis results from a combination of inherited or acquired genetic predispositions coupled with glandular injury secondary to ingested compounds such as ethanol, prior mechanical injury, or injury secondary to other significant illness. The disease process leads to fibrosis, which yields mass effect and obstructs ductal drainage. Chronic inflammatory changes result in pain syndromes caused by directly injuring nerves and through humoral release of pain neurotransmitters. Ductal obstruction causes conditions to persist that provide a positive feedback loop for continued glandular injury (Martin RF and Marion MD. Surg Clinc N Am 2007;87:1461-75).

The old controversy "resection or drainage" is probably now irrelevant. Both have established roles and probably best results are achieved by a combination of both. Chronic pancreatitis is such a complex and variegated disease that there is never a single procedure that would achieve goals in all patients. Therefore, it is important to understand that the choice of surgery has to be individualized to address the pathological change in each patient. However, ultimately it is the surgeons experience and an operative strategy that is slightly modified for every patient that is going to achieve the best possible results and which is what would be ultimately an ideal or somewhat close to ideal procedure for chronic pancreatitis. However, most of the operative procedures described in this monogram need a larger series of treated patients to be followed to adopt a definitive and probably better future strategy for managing this complex problem. However, the good news for a pancreatic surgeon is that operative management can be performed with low mortality and acceptable morbidity. Surgical treatment can provide good pain control, return patients to work, and achieve a satisfactory quality of life in the majority of patients. Longterm mortality is high in a subset of patients (Schnelldorfer T *et al.* J Am Coll Surg 2007;204:1039-1047). Latest literature suggests the role of oral pancreatic enzyme supplmentation and dietary modification in improving digestive tract function in people with chronic pancreatitis (The *Medifocus Guidebook on Chronic Pancreatitis*, 123 pages; last updated June 21, 2011).

8. Acknowledgement

- Prof G Q Peer who always trusted and believed in me and infused confidence in me at critical junctures.
- Prof Khursheed Alam Wani -Head Dept of Surgery at SKIMS who always encouraged and facilitated my research work and kept on appreciating my good work at all junctures.
- Prof Nisar A Chowdri who always trusted and believed in me for quality work.
- Dr Sameer H Naqash, Dr Ajaz A Malik and Dr Rouf A Wani, Dr Mubashir A Shah and Dr Munir A Wani my dearest colleagues in the department who always stood by me morally and professionally during the study period.
- Mr Farooq A Nadaf for always sincerely executing my computer work with lots of zeal and commitment.
- My revered parents for their love, affection and blessing.
- My beloved wife Nighat who is a big psychological, emotional and moral support for my all academic work and my sweet kids Shaheem and Liqa who always bear with me in my hours of toil at the cost of their time.
- My dearest students who always gave me lots of love and respect and made me to do better.

9. References

Augusto JB, Niederhuber JE. (1998). The pancreas. In: Niederhuber JE, Dunwoody SL, editors. Fundamentals of surgery.1st ed. Stanford: Appleton and Lange; p. 375-89.

Barret O, Bowers WF. (1957). Total pancreatectomy for relapsing and calcinosis of pancreas. *USAF Med J*, 8:1037-41.

Bartlet MK, Nardi GL. (1960). Treatment of recurrent pancreatitis by transduodenal sphincterotomy and exploration of the pancreatic duct. *New Engl J Med*, 262:642-8.

Bagley FH, *et al.* (1981). Sphincterotomy or sphincteroplasty in the treatment of pathological mild pancreatitis. *Am J Surg*, 141:418-21.

Bockmann DE, *et al.* (1988). Analysis of nerves in chronic pancreatitis. *Gastroenterology*, 94:1459-69.

Buchler M *et al.* (1995). Randomized trail of duodenum preserving pancreatic head resection versus pylorus preserving Whipple in chronic pancreatitis. *Am J Surg*, 169:65-70.

Bapat RD, *et al.* (1997) Modified Partington procedure for pancreaticojejunostomy in chronic pancreatitis. *Indian J Gastroenterol*, 16(3):122-5

Beger HG, *et al.*(1999). Duodenum preserving head resection in chronic pancreatitis changes the natural course of the disease. A single centre 26 year experience. *Ann Surg*, 230:512-23.

Blondet JJ, et al. (2007).The Role of Total Pancreatectomy and Islet Autotransplantation for Chronic Pancreatitis. *Surgical Clinics of North America*, 87(6): 1477-1501.

Copenhagen pancreatitis study.(1981). An interim report from a prospective epidemiological multicentre study. *Scand J Gastroenterol*, 16:305-12.

Campanale RP, *et al.* (1985). Reliability and sensitivity of frozen section pancreatic biopsy. *Arch Surg*, 12:283-8.

Catalano MF, *et al.* (1998). Prospective evaluation of endoscopic ultrasonography and secretin test in the diagnosis of chronic pancreatitis. *Gastrointest Endoscop*, 48(1):11-7 [medline].

Clain JE, Pearson RK. (1999). Diagnosis of chronic pancreatitis: is a gold standard necessary? *Surg Clin North Am*, 79:829-46.

Duval MK. (1954). Caudal pancreaticojejunostomy for chronic relapsing pancreatitis. *Ann Surg*, 140:775-85.

Doubilet H, Mulholland JH. (1956). Eight year study of pancreatitis and sphincterotomy. *J Am Med Assoc*, 160:521-8.

Dionigi R, *et al.* (2006). Chirugia con CD ROM,Pancreas, 14,vol(1-2):705-706.

Ebbehoj N, *et al.* (1984). Pancreatic tissue pressure in chronic obstructive pancreatitis. *Scand J Gastroenterol*, 19:1066-8.

Easter DW, Cushieri A. (1991). Total pancreatectomy with preservation of the duodenum and pylorus for chronic pancreatitis.*Ann Surg*, 214:575-80.

Evans TD, *et al.* (1997). Outcome of surgery for chronic pancreatitis.*Br J Surg*,84:624-9.

EUS-Based Criteria For The Diagnosis Of Chronic Pancreatitis: The Rosemont Classification. ScienceDaily ,June 29, 2009; American Society for Gastrointestinal Endoscopy.

Fery CF, *et al.* (1989). Pancreatic resection for chronic pancreatitis. *Surg Clin North Am*, 69:499-528.

Frey CF, Ho HS. (1997). Distal pancreatectomy in chronic pancreatitis. In: Trede M, Carter DC, editors. Surgery of the pancreas.New York: Churchill Livingstone; p. 347-5.

Frey CF. (1999). The surgical management of chronic pancreatitis. The Frey procedure. *Adv Surg*, 32:41-85.

Grimm H, *et al.* (1989). New modalities for treating chronic pancreatitis. *Endoscopy*, 21:70-4.

Grenlee HB, *et al.* (1990). Long term results of side to side pancreaticojejunostomy. *World J Surg*,14:70-6.

Gagner M, Pomp A. (1994). Laparoscopic Pylorus Preserving Pancreatoduodenectomy. *Surg Endosc*, 8(5):408-10.

Govil S, Imrie CG. (1999). Value of splenic preservation during distal pancreatectomy for chronic pancreatitis. *Br J Surg*, 86(7):895-8.

Hinshaw DB, *et al.* (1981). Islet auto-transplantation after pancreatectomy for chronic pancreatitis with a new method of islet preparation. *Am J Surg*, 42:118.
Hiraoka T, *et al.* (1986). A new surgical approach for treatment of pain in chronic pancreatitis: complete deneravation of the pancreas. *Am J Surg*, 152:459.
Izbicki JR, *et al.* (1995). Duodenum preserving resection of the head of the pancreas in chronic pancreatitis. *Ann Surg*, 221(4):350-8.
Izbicki JR, *et al.* (1998). Longitudinal V shaped excision of the ventral pancreas for small duct disease in severe pancreatitis. *Ann Surg*, 227(2):213-24.
Jordan GL, *et al.* (1977). Current status of pancreaticojejunostomy in the management of chronic pancreatitis. *Am J Surg*, 133:46-550.
Kore M, *et al.* (1994). Chronic pancreatitis is associated with increased concentration of Epidermal growth factor receptor, Transforming growth factor and phispholipase C gamma. *Gut*, 35:1468-73.
Knoeful WT, *et al.* (2002). Optimizing surgical therapy for chronic pancreatitis. *Pancreatology*, 2:379-85.
Leger L, *et al.* (1974). Five to 25 years follow up after surgery for chronic pancreatitis in 148 patients. *Ann Surg*, 180:180-91.
Lerut JP, *et al.* (1984). Pancreaticoduodenal resection surgical experience and evaluation of risk factors in 103 patients. *Ann Surg*, 1999:432-7.
Lowenfels AB, *et al.* (1993). Pancreatitis and the risk of pancreatic cancer. International pancreatitis study group. *New Engl J Med*, 328:1433-7.
Laukoisch PG. (1993). Function tests in the diagnosis of chronic pancreatitis. Critical evaluation. *Int J Pancreatol*, 14(1):9-20.
Lin Y, *et al.* (2003). Nationwide epidemiological survey of chronic pancreatitis in Japan. *J Gastroenterol*, 35: 136-41.
Moreno-Gonzales I, *et al.* (1982). Biliary and pancreaticoduodenal division by means of an isolated jejunal loop. *Br J Surg*, 69: 254.
Mallet Guy PA. (1983). Late and very late results of resection of the nervous system in chronic relapsing pancreatitis. *Am J Surg*, 145:234.
Maras WB, *et al.* (1995). Randomized trial of duodenum preserving pancreatic head resection versus pylorus preserving Whipple in chronic pancreatitis. *Ann Surg*, 221(4):350-8.
Modlin IM, *et al.* (2002). The evolution of pancreatic therapy. International Hepato-pancreato-biliary Association, Indian chapter, single theme conference, p. 32-46.
Makarewicz W, *et al.* (2003). Quality of life improvement after videothoracoscopic in chronic pancreatitis patients: case control study. *World J Surg*, 27:906-11.
Martin RF & Marion MD. (2007). Resectional therapy for chronic panreatitis. *Surg Clinc N Am*, 87:1461-75.
Puestow CB, Gillesby WT. (1958). Retrograde surgical drainage of pancreas for chronic pancreatitis. *Arch Surg*, 76:898-906.
Partington RF, Rochelle REL. (1960). Modified Puestow procedure for retrograde drainage of the pancreatic duct. *Ann Surg*, 152:1037-42.
Pain JA, Knight MJ. (1989). Pancreaticogastrostomy: the preferred operation for pain. Pancreaticogastrostomy for chronic pancreatitis. *Am J Surg*, 157:315-7.
Rumpf KD, Pichlmayr R. (1983). Eirie method Zur Chirurgischen behind lung der chronischen pancreatitis. *Die transduodenal pancreaticoplaslik. Chirurg*, 54:722-7.

Rossi RL, *et al.* (1986). Segmental pancreatic auto-transplantation with pancreatic ductal occlusion after near total pancreatic resection for chronic pancreatitis. *Ann Surg,* 203:626.

Rossi RL, *et al.* (1987). Pancreaticoduodenectomy in the management of chronic pancreatitis. Arch Surg, 122:416-20.

Robles-Diaz G, *et al.* (1990). Chronic pancreatitis in Mexico city. *Pancreas,* 5:479-83.

Reila A, *et al.* (1992). Increasing incidence of pancreatic cancer among women in Olmsted Country, Minnesota, 1940 through 1988. *Mayo Clin Proc,* 67:839-45.

Ramesh H, Augustine P. (1992). Surgery in tropical pancreatitis: analysis of risk factors. *Br J Surg,* 79:544-9.

Sarles H. Pancreatitis. In: Symposium of Marseille 1963. Basel, Switzerland: Karger; 1965.

Shires III GT, *et al.* (1986). Denervated splenopancreatic flap for chronic pancreatitis. *Ann Surg,* 203:568.

Sarner M, Cotton PB. (1984). Definitions of pancreatitis. *Gut,* 24:756-9.

Sota JA, *et al.* (1995). MR cholangiopancreatography findings on 3D fast spin echo imaging. *AJR Am J Roentgenol,* 165(6):1397-401 [medline].

Seiler CA, et al. (2005). Randomized clinical trial of pylorus-preserving duodenopancreatectomy *versus* classical Whipple resection—long term results. British Journal of Surgery,92 (5) : 547–556,

Schnelldorfer T, *et al.* (2007). Operative management of Chronic Pancreatitis:Long term results in 372 patients. *J Am Coll Surg,* 204:1039-1047.

Samuel M, et al. (Oct 2010). Laparoscopic and da Vinci Robot-Assisted Total Pancreaticoduodenectomy and Intraportal Islet Autotransplantation: Case Report of a Definitive Minimally Invasive Treatment of Chronic Pancreatitis.Pancreas; 39(7): 1109-1111.

Traverso LW, Longmire WP. (1978). Preservation of pylorus in pancreaticoduodenectomy. *Surg Gynecol Obstet,* 156:581-6.

Traverso LW, Kozarek RA. (1997). Pancreaticoduodenectomy for chronic pancreatitis: anatomical selection criteria and subsequent long term outcome analysis. *Ann Surg,* 226:429-38.

The Medifocus Guidebook on Chronic Pancreatitis (123 pages; last updated June 21, 2011).

Udani PM, *et al.* (1999). Choice of surgical procedure for chronic pancreatitis. <http/bhj.org/journal/1999:4102>.

Uranues S, et al. (2006). Laparoscopic resection of the pancreatic tail with splenic preservation.The American Journal of Surgery;192(2): 257-261

Watson K. (1944). Carcinoma of ampulla of Vater: successful radical resection. *Br J Surg,* 31:368-73.

Withigen J, Frey CF. (1974). Islet concentration in the head, body, tail and uncinate process of the pancreas. *Ann Surg,* 179:412-8.

Warren WD, *et al.* (1984). A denervated pancreatic flap for control of chronic pain in pancreatitis. *Surg Gynecol Obstet* 1984;159:581-6.

Wani NA, et al. (2007). Is any surgical procedure ideal for chronic pancreatitis. *International Journal of Surgery,* 5:45-56.

Yasuda H, *et al.* (1990). Resection of the head of the pancreas with preservation of biliary tract and duodenum. *J Biliary Tract Pancreas,* 11:967-73.

Yakshe P. (2004). Chronic pancreatitis, e-medicine article last updated August 25.

7

Total Pancreatectomy and Islet Autotransplantation for Chronic Pancreatitis

David E.R. Sutherland[1,2] et al.*
[1]*Schulze Diabetes Institute,*
[2]*Department of Surgery,*
USA

1. Introduction

Total pancreatectomy (TP) or near-total pancreatectomy with islet auto-transplantation (IAT) to treat chronic pancreatitis (CP) was first done in 1977 at the University of Minnesota (UMN) (Sutherland et al., 1978). The idea evolved from a desire to compare metabolic outcomes between islet autografts in pancreatectomized individuals, who could not reject their graft, and islet allografts done to treat type 1 diabetes, to understand why the latter failed (was it for technical or immunologic reasons? (Najarian et al., 1979). The main rationale from the beginning, however, was to relieve the pain of CP in patients in whom other measures had failed (Morrow et al., 1984), and to preserve beta (ß)-cell mass and insulin secretory capacity in order to prevent or minimize the otherwise inevitable surgical diabetes (Blondet et al., 2007; Najarian et al., 1980). Surgical diabetes is often described as brittle (Pezzilli, 2006), in part because of erratic food absorption from exocrine deficiency (Stauffer et al., 2009), but there are reports where metabolic parameters after TP are similar to patients with type 1 diabetes (Fujino et al., 2009).

Although IATs have been done with pancreatic resections for premalignant (Sakata et al., 2008) and malignant (Forster et. al , 2004) neoplasias, as well as for acute relapsing pancreatitis (ARP) before evolution to CP occurs (Sutherland et al., 2011a), the major application of TP-IAT has been in patients who have CP and intractable pain (Blondet et al., 2007; Carlson et al., 2007; Dong et al., 2011; Hermann et al., 2010; Matsumoto, 2011; Onaca et al., 2007; Ong et al., 2009; Robertson, 2010a; Sutherland et al., 2011a). TP, with or without (Behrman & Mulloy, 2006; Casadei et al., 2010a; Casadei et al., 2010b; Fujino Y et al., 2009; Gruessner et al., 2008; Heidt et al., 2007; Janot et al., 2010; Muller et al., 2007; Mullhaupt & Ammann, 2010; Stauffer et al., 2009) IAT, may appear to be a radical treatment, but for the CP patients in whom it is done, the alternative is even more radical: persistent pain and/or

---

* Melena Bellin[1,3], Juan J. Blondet[2], Greg J. Beilman[2], Ty B. Dunn[2], Srinath Chinnakotla[2,3], Timothy L. Pruett[2], Martin L. Freeman[4], A.N. Balamurugan[1], Barbara Bland[2], David Radosevich[2] and Bernhard J. Hering[1,2]
[1]*Schulze Diabetes Institute, University of Minnesota, Minneapolis, MN, USA*
[2]*Department of Surgery, University of Minnesota, Minneapolis, MN, USA*
[3]*Department of Pediatrics, University of Minnesota, Minneapolis, MN, USA*
[4]*Department of Medicine, University of Minnesota, Minneapolis, MN, USA*

lifetime narcotic use (Ahmad et al., 2005; Braganza et al., 2011; Gachago & Draganov, 2008; Mullhaupt & Ammann, 2010). Thus, an appreciation of the spectrum of the disease, the inconsistency in correlation between imaging and gross and microscopic pathology results and the degree of pain, and the various mechanisms by which CP causes pain are relevant for patient selection and for interpretation of the outcomes in the TP-IAT series reviewed here.

2. Brief review of chronic pancreatitis and treatment options

CP is characterized by progressive, irreversible damage to the pancreas, with varying degrees of inflammation, fibrosis, ductal alteration, exocrine atrophy, and secondary involvement of the islets of Langerhans (Braganza et al., 2011). The clinical manifestations also vary as to the degree of pain, maldigestion from loss of exocrine function, and occurrence of diabetes. Although lost exocrine function can be managed with oral pancreatic enzyme supplements, and diabetes, if it occurs, with insulin, the hallmark of CP is pain, often intractable and debilitating. Pain is the main symptom toward which therapies are directed, all with significant failure rates (Gachago & Draganov, 2008).

The acute and chronic forms of pancreatitis are not totally distinguishable. They have overlapping risk factors and share a common pathogenic origin as a pancreatic autodigestive process. Additionally, they each may manifest as an initial episode of abdominal pain, with elevation of serum amylase and lipase, and with similar nonspecific inflammatory changes. CP is likely the result of progressive pancreatic damage after recurrent episodes of pancreatic necro-inflammation. The sentinel acute pancreatitis event (SAPE) hypothesis (Schneider & Whitcomb, 2002), postulates that the sentinel event is a pancreatic injury that makes the gland particularly vulnerable, in the recovery phase, to additional insults such as alcohol, metabolic, and oxidative stresses. ARP may evolve to CP; patients who are initially pain free between episodes may begin to have underlying interval pain and may cease having episodes altogether. Even one episode of acute pancreatitis may be followed by evolution to CP, or CP may occur without a history of an identifiable episode of acute pancreatitis. Whatever the trigger, progression of CP to end-stage fibrosis occurs at different rates in different people, and can be caused by different mechanisms (Etemad & Whitcomb, 2001).

Traditionally, alcohol abuse has been thought to be the cause of most cases of CP, but this perception may not be correct. Indeed, in the first 135 cases of TP-IAT for CP at UMN, only 16% were attributed to alcohol, and 60% were idiopathic (Jie et al., 2005); in more recent cases (Sutherland et al., 2011b) fewer are classified as idiopathic and more as genetic in origin because of the identification of genes associated with CP as well as pancreatic cancer (Braganza et al., 2011). In the series at the University of Cincinnati, only 14% of the cases of CP were attributed to alcohol (Ahmad et al., 2005; Sutton et al., 2010). Cigarette smoking is also a major risk factor for CP (Maisonneuve et al., 2005; Talamini et al, 1999). Well-defined inherited germline mutations also can cause CP in families (Whitcomb, 2000). Hereditary pancreatitis once was thought to be rare, diagnosed only when other family members are affected. The identification of PRSS1, SPINK1, and CFTR mutations in patients with so-called idiopathic CP, however, indicates that genetic risk factors are much more common than originally envisioned (Braganza et al., 2011; Witt et al., 2011).

These mutations have both autosomal-dominant and recessive patterns of inheritance with variable penetration and may be influenced by certain modifier genes and environmental factors. The discovery of SPINK1 mutations in various types of CP, such as tropical calcific, alcoholic, and autoimmune pancreatitis, blurs the borders between the particular CP subtypes Other risk factors for CP include biliary lithiasis, anatomical variants like annular pancreas or divisum, hypertriglyceridemia, hypercalcemia, sphincter of Oddi dysfunction, and trauma (Ahmad et al., 2005; Braganza et al., 2011; Jie et al., 2005; Witt et al., 2011;). The key histopathologic features of CP, regardless of the etiology, are varying degrees (Kobayashi et al., 2010; Kobayashi et al., 2011) and combinations of pancreatic fibrosis, acinar atrophy, acute and chronic inflammation, and distorted or blocked ducts (Braganza et al., 2011).

The diagnosis of CP is based mainly on symptoms, imaging studies, and supporting laboratory tests. In certain patients, the diagnosis can be surprisingly difficult, especially in those who have early or mild small-duct or minimal-change variants (Braganza et al., 2011; Layer et al., 1994; Walsh et al., 1992). Serum amylase and lipase levels typically are elevated during attacks early on but might be normal in later phases with progressive destruction of the gland. Imaging studies include (CT), endoscopic retrograde cholangiopancreatography (ERCP) (which is associated with a risk of precipitating pancreatitis), magnetic resonance cholangiopancreatography (MRCP), and endoscopic ultrasound (EUS) (Kahl et al., 2002). Although all of the studies can detect ductal and textural abnormalities, the specificity and sensitivity of each in diagnosing CP are not defined well, given the difficulty of obtaining histopathologic correlation, and when it was obtained in a large series at UMN, the correlation was poor with CP clearly present in patients with minimal findings on the imaging studies (Vega-Peralta et al., 2011a; Vega-Peralta et al., 2011b).

The treatment of patients who have CP is focused on mitigating their unrelenting or recurring abdominal pain (Braganza et al., 2011; Gachago & Draganov, 2008; Kobayashi et al., 2010). Patients who imbibe alcohol or smoke should stop. Pancreatic enzyme supplementation may help. Non-narcotic analgesics should be tried first, but many need narcotic analgesics; patient comfort takes precedence over concerns of addiction (Ahmad et.al., 2006; Andren-Sandberg et al., 2002; Fasanella et al., 2007). Some patients need escalating doses, with the addition of fentanyl patches or even parenteral administration. Celiac ganglion blocks, percutaneous or endoscopic, can be tried but rarely give permanent pain relief, if any at all, and transient responses often cannot be repeated (Warshaw et al., 1998). Patients who require narcotic analgesics, with or without complete relief, are candidates for invasive procedures in an attempt to remove or modify the root cause of the pain. The general progression is from the least to the most invasive procedure, depending on the response.

Pain in CP occurs with or without ductal obstruction. When obstruction, increased intra-ductal pressure, or a dilated duct can be demonstrated, efforts should be made to relieve the obstruction. If pain persists or recurs, then the next step is pancreatic resection. Because previous surgical drainage procedures (Puestow or Berger or Frey) compromise islet yield if a subsequent TP-IAT is done (Bellin et al., 2010a; Jie et al., 2005; Sutherland et al., 2011b), the current UMN paradigm is to do any indicated drainage procedures endoscopically only (Sutherland et al., 2011b). Then, if the endoscopic drainage is unsuccessful, the authors proceed to resection rather than surgical drainage. Although two randomized trials of highly selected subgroups of patients who had severe CP cases showed that primary surgical drainage had a better chance of relieving pain than endoscopic drainage (Cahen et al., 2007; Dite et al., 2003), most gastroenterologists, because it is minimally invasive, advocate an initial trial of endoscopic therapy in an attempt to relieve pain in patients who have a dilated duct, stricture, or pancreatic stones (Wilcox & Varadarajulu, 2006). If endoscopic drainage fails, there is little evidence that surgical drainage will be successful in relieving pain. As primary therapy, each approach has a relatively high failure rate; pain persisted in 68% of patients who had endoscopic and 25% who had surgical drainage in the study by Cahen and colleagues (Cahen et al., 2007). Even in those who have initial relief following either endoscopic or surgical drainage, it may not be sustained longer than 5 years (Braganza et al., 2011).

The ideal CP candidates for endoscopic drainage procedures have a focal proximal stricture associated with upstream dilation of the pancreatic duct, or relatively small burden of main pancreatic duct stones that is amenable to extraction with or without extracorporeal shock wave lithotripsy, or a pseudocyst. Endoscopic therapy most often is successful in patients who have moderate disease. Successful treatment of strictures requires aggressive therapy, with repeated dilations and stenting in hope that the stricture resolves. There is wide variability in expertise, aggressiveness, and conceptual approaches to endoscopic therapy, which may influence outcomes (Fasanella et al., 2007; Wilcox & Varadarajulu, 2006). Although the complication rate of endoscopic therapy is relatively low, acute episodes of pancreatitis can occur after sphincterotomy and stent placement, and in some patients, the underlying pain becomes worse; such patients are prime candidates for resection, including TP-IAT.

Pancreas resection is indicated in CP patients who have small-duct disease or those in whom endoscopic drainage fail, ideally with an IAT but many centers do or have done TP without an IAT (Behrman & Mulloy, 2006; Casadei et al., 2010a; Casadei et al., 2010b; Fujino Y et al., 2009; Gruessner et al., 2008; Janot et al., 2010; Muller et al., 2007; Stauffer et al., 2009). A TP is the most likely operation to relieve pain, and for CP patients who are already diabetic, there is little reason not to do it. For non-diabetic CP patients, a TP-IAT reduces but does not eliminate the risk of surgical diabetes. Thus, a case can be made for partial resection (usually a Whipple operation, but a distal pancreatectomy for the rare case with a mid-duct stricture and CP of the body and tail only). If pain is not relieved by a partial resection, a completion pancreatectomy with IAT can be done subsequently (Sutherland et al., 2011b).

Patients tend to be referred for resection late in the course of CP, often with a pain history of years, and many opt for TP rather than a partial resection, wanting the best chance at pain relief without the risk of reoperation. TP-IAT done early in the course of CP avoids the complications of chronic narcotic use and gives the best chance at a high islet yield to prevent or minimize post-pancreatectomy diabetes (Bellin et al., 2010a; Kobayashi et al., 2010; Kobayashi et al., 2011; Sutherland et al., 2011b; Takita et al., 2010).

The authors' experience indicates that TP with preservation of β-cell mass by immediate isolation and intraportal transplantation of islets from the excised pancreas should be considered as a primary surgical option for patients who have painful CP refractory to less invasive procedures (Blondet et al., 2007; Jie et al., 2005; Sutherland et al., 2011b; Wahoff et.al., 1995a). The main criterion for success of the islet autograft per se is whether insulin independence is maintained or surgical diabetes made milder. The overall outcome, however, depends as much on the clinical response as on the metabolic results, specifically whether the patient's pain is reduced or eliminated, narcotic analgesics withdrawn, and the quality of life (QOL) improved (Bellin et al., 2010b; Bellin et al., 2011b; Bellin et al., 2011c; Billings et al., 2011; Rafael et al., 2008; Sutton et al., 2010).

3. Historical context

The first patient in the UMN series (and the world) to undergo an IAT after pancreatectomy (Sutherland et al., 1978), in 1977, remained insulin-independent and pain-free until she died 6 years later of causes not related to her operation (Farney et al., 1991). This case proved that a viable islet preparation could be made from a freshly excised human pancreas. It also showed that the previous failures with islet allografts were caused either by low viability or poor preservation of deceased donor pancreases, or rejection (Najarian et al., 1977) .

As of mid-2011 the UMN IAT experience includes more than 400 cases (Sutherland et al., 2011b). The outcomes in the UMN series have been periodically published (Farney et al., 1991; Farney et al., 1998; Gores et al., 1992; Gruessner et al., 2004; Hering et al., 2004; Jie et al., 2005; Morrow et al., 1984; Najarian et al., 1979; Najarian et al., 1980; Najarian et al., 1977; Robertson et al., 2001; Sutherland et al., 1978; Sutherland et al., 1980a; Sutherland et al., 2004a; Sutherland et al., 2009a; Sutherland et al., 2009b; Sutherland et al., 2011b; Wahoff et al., 1995a; Wahoff et al., 1995b), including in children (Bellin et al., 2007; Bellin et al., 2008; Bellin et al., 2010a; Bellin & Sutherland, 2010; Bellin et al., 2010b; Bellin et al., 2011b; Wahoff et.al., 1996).

Shortly after the initial report on IAT from the UMN more than 30 years ago (Sutherland et al., 1978), a few other centers also did IAT after total or partial pancreatectomy (Cameron et al., 1981; Fontana et al., 1994; Hinshaw et al., 2011; Mehigan et al., 1980; Mehigan et al., 1980; Memsic et al., 1984; Mirkovitch et al., 1981; Toledo-Pereyra et al., 1984; Traverso et al.,1981) though because they were done without anticoagulation complications of the IAT occurred at some centers (Mehigan et al., 1980; Memsic et al., 1984; Toledo-Pereyra et al., 1984), but inexplicably not at others (Fontana et al., 1994; Hinshaw et al., 2011; Valente et al., 1986). Later several center began programs with low complication rates because of lessons learned from the others (Blondet et al., 2007). To date, more than 30 are known to have done IAT, nearly all by embolization of the isolated islets to the liver by means of the portal vein (Fig. 1). The world literature as of 2011 contains reports of about 700 IATs, including the 400 UMN cases cited previously and those done elsewhere (Ahmad et al., 2005; Argo et al., 2008; Clayton et al., 2003; Dixon et al., 2008; Farkas & Pap, 1997; Garcea et al., 2009; Jindal et al., 1998; Oberholzer et al., 2000; Rodriguez et al., 2003; Sarbu et al., 2005; Sutton et al., 2010; Takita et al., 2010; Takita et al., 2011a; Teuscher et al., 1998; Watkins et al., 2003; Webb et al., 2008; White et al., 1998; White et al., 2001;)[2622]. After UMN, the next largest series are at the University of Cincinnati (more than 100) and the University of Leicester (more than 60).

For historical completeness, segmental pancreatic auto-transplantation is mentioned as another method for preserving β-cell mass after pancreatic resection (Fukushima et al., 1994 Hogle & Recemtsma, 1978; Rossi et al., 1986). The first such case was done around the time of the first IAT (Hogle & Recemtsma , 1978). This approach appears to have been used less frequently than IAT; indeed, no reports have appeared in the literature on segmental pancreas auto-transplants for the past decade.

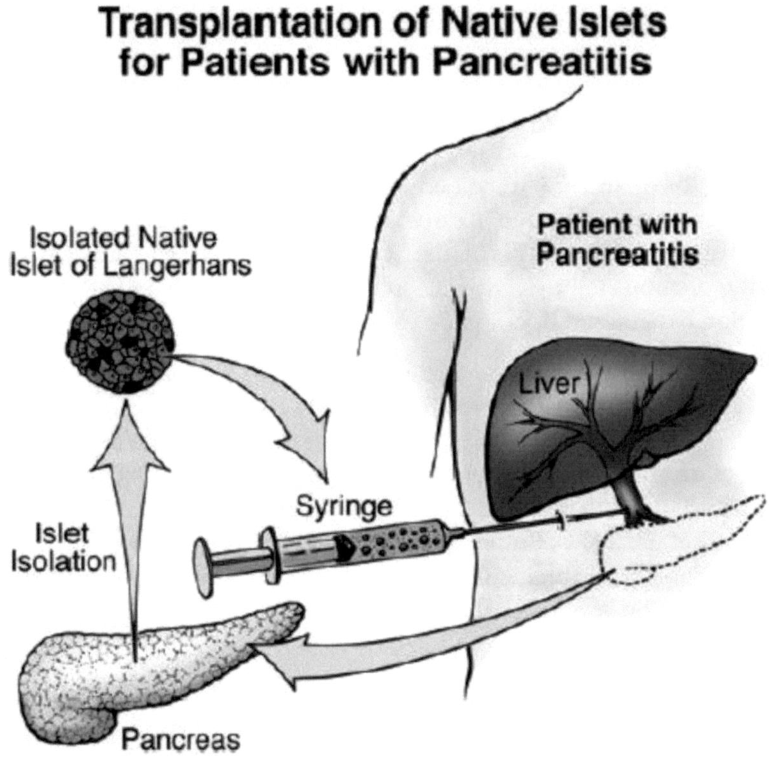

Fig. 1. Sequence of events to preserve beta-cell mass in patients undergoing a total pancreatectomy for benign disease. The resected pancreas is dispersed by collagenase digestion followed by islet isolation. Autologous islets then are embolized to the patient's liver by means of the portal vein (from Blondet et al 2007).

4. Patient selection and pain syndrome

The severity of the gross morphologic changes associated with pancreatitis, as detected by imaging studies, do not correlate necessarily with the degree of pain the patient is experiencing (Noh & Wallace , 2006; Sahai et al., 1998). Nor do normal or near normal imaging studies rule out CP (Gupta et al., 2007; Vega-Peralta et al., 2011a; Vega-Peralta et al., 2011b). Minimal change CP was first described by Walsh and colleagues (Walsh et al., 1992) in patients who had severe abdominal pain with minimal gross morphologic changes but clear histopathologic changes in the gland, with resolution of pain in most patients following pancreatectomy. Layer and colleagues (Layer et al., 1994), also described two forms of CP: early-onset CP, where pain precedes by years the development of gross pathologic changes, and late-onset CP, where gross changes are already detectable by the time the patient has pain. These two papers were published before the EUS era.

Ideally, EUS should allow minimal change CP to be detected, but because it is standard to require that five of the nine features tested for on EUS (hyperechoic parenchymal foci, strands, hypoechoic lobules, cysts, main duct irregularity, ductal dilation, hyperechoic duct walls, visible side branches, and calcifications or stones) be present for a diagnosis of CP to be made to avoid overcalling (Sahai et al., 1998), the minimal change variety may be present but not diagnosed (Vargas et al., 2001; Vega-Peralta et al., 2011a).

At UMN we have correlated EUS findings (classified using 9 standard criteria) with resected pancreas histopathology in 50 patients with minimal change chronic pancreatic (MCCP) (no calicifications in the pancreas on CT scan) out of 141 undergoing TP-IAT from 1/2008 through 7/2010 because of severe abdominal pain thought secondary to CP (Vega-Peralta et al., 2011a; Vega-Peralta et al., 2011b). MCCP was defined histologically when fibrosis, atrophy or inflammation was found in at least 1 biopsy. . Of pts with histologically confirmed MCCP, 27/45(60%) had ≥4/9criteria on EUS. 18/21(85%) pts with ≤3EUS criteria and 4/5(80%) pts with 0/9EUS criteria had MCCP by histopathology. 2/29(7%) pts with ≥4/9EUS criteria had normal histology. Negative predictive value of a normal EUS was 38%. Positive predictive value of abnormal EUS at ≥6criteria was 72%. Correlation between EUS and histology of MCCP is poor in pts undergoing TP-IAT. This study showed that normal or nearly normal EUS cannot exclude MCCP, and abnormal EUS alone is probably not sufficient for the diagnosis unless ≥6 criteria are present. The clinical syndrome is important in MCCP. If it fits the pain pattern seen in CP, treatment, including TP-IAT, should be based on clinical rather than imaging criteria.

Further support for the contention that the current criteria, designed to prevent over-diagnosing CP on EUS (Sahai et al., 1998), may under-diagnose comes from Chong and colleagues (Chong et al., 2007)at the Medical University of South Carolina. They found that a threshold of three criteria gave the best balance between sensitivity (83%) and specificity (80%) for correlation of EUS findings with histological CP. Thus, patients who have an abdominal pain syndrome who have any one of the nine features consistent with CP on EUS may indeed have the disease, probably in the minimal change category. The authors know of no report in the literature that correlates the severity of pain and the morphologic findings of radiologic or pathologic studies.

The pain of pancreatitis is multifactorial (Di Sebastiano et al., 1997; Di Sebastiano et al., 2004; Keith et al., 1985;). Even when there is increased ductal pressure, it is not necessarily the cause of the pain (Manes et al., 1994), and pain in patients who have CP exists in the absence of increased ductal pressure. Indeed microscopic pathology with intrinsic neuritis had the best correlation in at least one study (Keith et al., 1985). Some patients have increased sensitivity to pain of central origin, perhaps explaining the symptoms in minimal-change CP (Buscher et al., 2006).

Thus, at UMN, the authors do TP-IAT in CP patients who have intractable pain, whether the gross morphologic changes detected in the pancreas are minimal or severe. It is almost always worth an attempt at islet isolation, because having even a small beta-cell mass is better than having none. Occasionally, and especially in CP patients who already have impaired glucose tolerance, the pancreas is such a small atrophic rock that the authors make a decision not to go to the expense and effort of an islet isolation that is almost certain to be ultra-low. In one center, imaging studies of the pancreas correlated with islet yield, being higher in those with MCCP (Takita et al., 2011b).

Patients who have ARP are also candidates for TP-IAT if their episodes are frequent, disruptive, and persist over time, even if they are pain-free between episodes (Sutherland et al., 2011b). Evolution of ARP into CP, where elevated levels of serum amylase and lipase cease but pain persists, is common and often misunderstood as meaning the pain is other than pancreatic. In non-diabetic patients requiring narcotics for their pain who have a history of ARP associated with even minimal criteria for CP on imaging studies, the authors recommend TP-IAT.

Some patients who have CP have diabetes when referred for surgical consultation. In such patients, the decision for resection is easy, especially when exocrine deficiency also exists. Most patients, however, are seen when diabetes does not exist and thus a TP must be undertaken with the acceptance of diabetes as a tradeoff for pain relief and for the chance to discontinue narcotics. If an IAT prevents diabetes, it is a bonus. When a TP is done for CP in a non-diabetic patient, however, an IAT to preserve ß-cell mass should be done whenever possible (Pezzilli, 2006).

5. Surgical resection considerations

During TP, the blood supply to the pancreas should be preserved as long as possible to minimize the detrimental effects of warm ischemia on the islets (Corlett & Scharp, 1998; Desai et al., 2011; Sutherland et al., 1980a; White et al., 2000a). To do so, never separate the distal pancreas from the splenic vessels. If the splenic vessels are ligated in the hilum, the spleen may survive on its collateral vessels, but usually it has to be taken. When the spleen is spared, there is a risk of variceal formation in the gastric veins draining the spleen leading to late intestinal bleeding, or splenomegaly that can be painful, so the authors leave it only if it retains an absolutely normal appearance after hilar ligation. It is possible to leave the entire blood supply to the pancreas intact, including the gastroduodenal artery as well as the splenic artery an vein until the pancreas and duodenum is totally mobalized and ready for resection (Desai et al., 2011).

At UMN, early IAT series included cases with the entire duodenum preserved (95% pancreatectomy), but the complication rate was actually lower in patients who had part of the duodenum or the entire duodenum resected (Farney et al., 1991). For the past 20 years, in some cases the authors have done a pylorus- and fourth portion-sparing partial duodenectomy when possible, with orthotopic reconstruction by means of duodenoduodenostomy and choledochoduodenostomy (Fig. 2). The history of this technique for pancreatic head resection or TP has recently been articulated (Farney & Sutherland, 2008).

This is just one method of reconstruction. The proximal duodenum can also be anastamosed to the first loop of jejunum distal to the ligament of Trietz with a choledochodudonestomy to the distal duodenum. If only the proximal dudoneum is spared then it can be

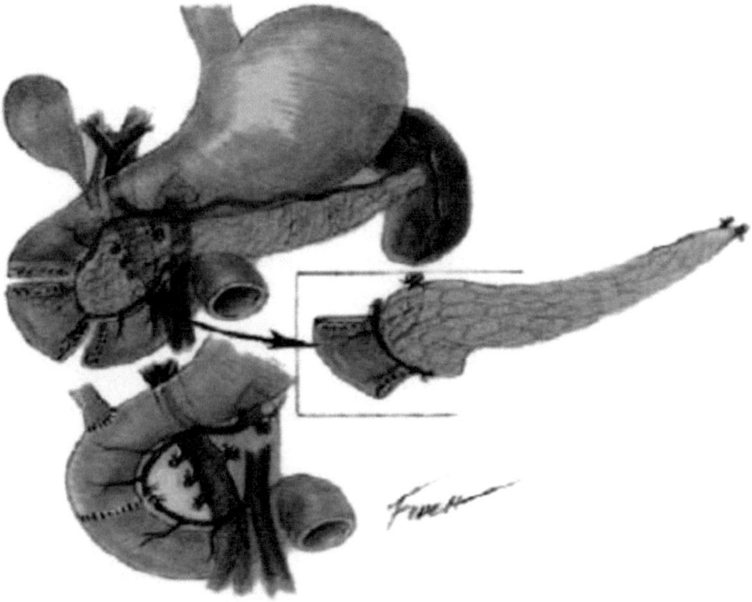

Fig. 2. Surgical technique for total pancreatectomy. Total pancreatectomy and pylorus- and distal-sparing duodenectomy with orthotopic reconstruction by means of duodenostomy and choledochoduodenostomy. (Adapted from Farney AC et al., 1991; with Copyright © 1991, Elsevier.)

anastaomosed to the jejunum with a choledochoduodenojejunostomy proximal to it. If the entire duodenum is removed so the pylorus is not spared, then a Roux-en-Y choldechojejunostomy is required to prevent bile reflux via the gastrojejunostomy. The author's current preference when the pylorus is spared is the second method described above but it is best to have all methods in one's armamentarium so one can adjust to the individual circumstances of the surgery

In others cases the proximal duodenum has been anastamosed end-to-side to the proximal jejunum just distal to the ligament of Trietz with a choledochoduodenostomy done to the distal (third or fourth portion) duodenum. Sparing the pylorus is done mainly to prevent bile reflux, but if it is or becomes incompetent enterogastric bile reflux can occur, and if symptomatic enough conversion to a Roux-en-y connection may be required by dividing the jejunum between the ligament of Trietz and the duodenojejunostomy and then performing a jejunojunostomy 45 cm or more distal to the duodenojejunostomy.

The technique used is surgeon's preference. Some members of our team always remove the entire duodenum with reconstruction via a Roux-en-y gastro- or duodenoo-jejunostomy and choledeochojejunostomy done so enterogastric bile reflux is not possible. With this method efforts to save the pylorus are unnecessary. The option of doing a cutaneous gastrostomy and feeding jejunostomy also exists, allowing for enteral rather than intravenous nutrition to be provided during the recovery period. Again, this is surgeon preference and can be individualized depending on the anticipation of recovery of bowel function. The impact of narcotic bowel syndrome, which many of these patients have, must also be taken into consideration (Grunkemeier et al., 2007).

There are many articles on surgical technique of TP (with or without IAT) and the complications there of and these should be read by all who perform such surgery (Behrman & Mulloy, 2006; Casadei et al., 2009; Casadei et al., 2010a; Casadei et al., 2010b; Fujino Y et al., 2009; Janot et al., 2010; Muller et al., 2007; Murphy et al., 2009; Parsaik et al., 2010; Simons et al., 2009; Stauffer et al., 2009). In addition, there are recent reports of pancretectomy done laproscopically, either hand assisted (Kitasato et al., 2011) or using the DaVinci Robotic Device (Giulianotti et al., 2009; Giulianotti et al., 2011), with the first TP-IAT for CP done at the University of Minnesota in 2008 (Marquez et al., 2010) .

There is also the option of trying preserve the spleen at the time of TP (Desai et al., 2011; Wahoff et al., 1995a). In order to preserve blood supply to the pancreas up until the minute it is removed to prevent ischemic injury to the islets, the splenic artery and vein are not taken at their origin and termination respectively until the pancreas is removed and they are left intact without separation from the pancreas. The splenic artery and vein can be ligated in the hilum of the spleen and the spleen than survives on its collateral circulation (short gastric vessels and gastroepiloic vessels) if at all, as originally described for living donors of segmental pancreas transplants (Sutherland, et al., 1980b). Although preserving the spleen gives a theoretical advantage in terms of fighting infection, in a series of TP without IAT done for a variety of reasons, there was no difference in complications and outcomes in the short term in those who underwent splenectomy and those in whom the spleen was preserved (Koukoutsis et al., 2007). In the early part of the TP-IAT series at the University of Minnesota efforts were made to save the spleen (Wahoff et al., 1995a), but the authors rarely do so now unless the collateral circulation is excellent (Sutherland et al., 2011b).

6. Metabolic considerations

In patients who have painful CP referred for resection, baseline metabolic studies to assess ß-cell function include fasting and postprandial glucose, baseline and stimulated C-peptide, and glycosylated hemoglobin levels. Patients who have CP often have symptoms of exocrine insufficiency (steatorrhea), but formal evaluation usually is not done. IAT candidates are counseled that exocrine deficiency may be made worse or induced by TP. Exocrine deficiency may be responsible for the more erratic blood sugar control in pancreatic diabetes than type 1 diabetes because of erratic absorption making the predicted insulin dose more difficult to calculate (Jahansouz et al., 2011; Robertson, 2010a; Robertson, 2010b). However, at least one group has reported that diabetic control after TP (for a variety of reasons) without IAT is equivalent to that of patients with type 1 diabetes in their clinic (Jethwa et al., 2006). Nevertheless, the metabolic control does not approach that achieved with an IAT after TP, whether insulin-independent or not (Bellin et al., 2009; Rajab et al., 2008).

Although the authors often try to spare the proximal and distal duodenum during TP, data from the bariatric literature suggest that there may be a metabolic benefit of duodenectomy. GLP-1, produced by L cells in the distal intestinal tract is a powerful incretin. Patients who have a Roux-en-Y gastric bypass have increased levels of GLP-1 with improvement in diabetes, results not seen after restrictive bariatric procedures (Greenway et al., 2002; le Roux et al., 2006). It is possible that complete duodenectomy at the time of TP would increase GLP-1 levels and mirror the positive impact on insulin sensitivity seen in the bariatric duodenal bypass patients, allowing a reduced islet mass to sustain insulin independence.

As far as metabolic studies after TP-IAT, largely focused on glycemic control and need or lack of need for exogenous insulin and the value of functioning islets even if the mass is insufficient for insulin-independence, many have been published (Ahmad et al., 2005; Bellin et al., 2008; Bellin et al., 2009; Berney et al, 2000; Farney et al., 1998; Jie et al., 2005; Jung et al., 2009; Kendall et al., 1997; Lee et al, 2005; Leone et al., 1998; Ngo et al., 2011; Pyzdrowski et al., 1992; Robertson et al., 2001; Robertson, 2010a; Sutherland et al., 2008; Teuscher et al., 1998).

Tight glucose control is desirable after IAT in order to prevent glucose toxicity to the islet as they engraft (Bellin et al., 2009) . Thus the authors usually employ an insulin-drip in the immediate postoperative period after TP-IAT until s transition is made to enteral feeding (Bellin et al., 2009; Sutherland et al., 2011b). A closed loop artificial endocrine pancreas insulin delivery device is another option to use in the early postoperative period to maintain euglycemia (Kobayashi et al., 2010).

7. Islet isolation and infusion considerations

In the United States, islet isolation must be done in a laboratory that meets all of the US Food and Drug Administration (FDA) criteria for processed tissue. Pancreatic surgery centers that do not have an islet isolation facility thus cannot offer IAT or must collaborate with a center that can process and return islets to the center of origin (Langer et al., 2004; Matsumoto, 2011; Rabkin et al., 1997; Rabkin et al., 1999).

After resection, the pancreatic duct is cannulated, and the pancreas is dispersed by collagenase digestion, using the modified Ricordi technique (Gores et al., 1992; Gruessner et al., 2004). At UMN, the authors do not purify preparations with a low tissue volume to maximize the islet yield (Gores & Sutherland, 1993) a situation often found in fibrotic pancreases (Balamurugan et al., 2011b). If the crude tissue digest exceeds 15 mL, the authors usually reduce the volume by purifying all or part of the islet preparation, so that embolization to the liver occurs without any undue rise in portal pressure (Casey et al., 2002; Robertson, 2001; Wilhelm et al., 2011). If portal pressure reaches 20 to 30 cm of water, the residual preparation can be dispersed freely in the peritoneal cavity or transplanted beneath the kidney capsule, or sub-mucosal layer of the stomach, in the hope that the islets engraft (Cameron JL et al., 1981; Wilhelm et al., 2011). The authors' current preference is to purify islets so that the tissue volume is reduced to an amount tolerated by the portal vein, without any undue rise in pressure, but not to the degree that a large number of islets have to be discarded or placed in alternative sites. Sometimes the authors do not purify a high volume digest, because a high percentage of the islets are mantled by, or not cleaved from, a surrounding rim of exocrine tissue, and we will lose most by purification (Wilhelm et al., 2011). In minimal change CP, islet yields are similar to what is obtained from deceased donor pancreases for islet allografts (Soltani et al., 2011b).

Several advances in islet isolation from diseased pancreases have been made in recent years by various techniques, including altering enzyme combinations in the digestion process (Anazawa et al., 2009; Balamurugan et al., 2011a; Balamurugan et al., 2011c) and other maneuvers (Matsumoto, 2011) such as altering the high density gradient process for purification (Soltani et al., 2011a). There is a clear relationship also to islet yield depending on the severity of the imaging changes of gross pancreatic morphology (Takita et al., 2010) and the severity of the histopathology in both adults (Kobayashi et al., 2011) and children (Kobayashi et al., 2010). In severely fibrotic pancreases of children, ductal neogenesis of islets may be seen (Soltani et al., 2011c), which in some but not all cases is associated with a high islet yield. However, in adults, the presences of nesidioblastosis on histopatholgy is associated with s a statistically lower islet yield than when this feature is absent, probably because its presence is indicative of islet loss from the CP stimulating neogenesis, but the response is inadequate or is itself met by destruction from the pancreatic inflammation and fibrosis (Kobayashi et al., 2011). Predicting islet yield in advance is difficult (Bellin et al., 2010a), but it is clear that prior surgical duct drainage procedures or distal resections compromise yield (Bellin et al., 2011a; Blondet et al., 2007; Jie et al., 2005; Sutherland et al., 2011b). Other factors, such as body mass index (BMI), may also play a role (Takita et al., 2011c). It might be expected that total islet yield is higher with higher BMI, but Taikta et al (Takita et al., 2011c) found that even the islet equivalents/kg were higher.

Clinical observations and animal studies indicate that the liver (by means of the portal vein) is the most efficient site for islet engraftment (Gray, 1990; Rajab et al., 2008; Wahoff et al., 1995a; Warnock et al. , 1983) . Other sites used, such as the renal capsule (Gray et al., 1988; Gray et al., 1989; Matarazzo et al., 2002; Vargas et al., 2001), spleen (Gray, 1990; Gustavson et al., 2005; Sutton et al., 1989), omentum (Ao et al., 1993; Gustavson et al., 2005) and peritoneal cavity (Wahoff et al., 1994a; Wahoff et al., 1994b) rarely have been associated with function of islet autografts in people (Fontana et al., 1994; White et al., 2000b) . A recent clinical case report from Sweden demonstrated function (C-peptide positive) of an intramuscular IAT in a 7 year old child undergoing TP for CP (Rafael et al., 2008). The islet yield was high (6400 IE/kg), an amount that usually results in insulin-independence in children if embolized to the liver via the portal vein (Bellin & Sutherland, 2010), suggesting that better islet function might have been achieved if the islets has been placed intra-hepatic.

At any site, the islets initially survive by nutrient diffusion. During this period, they have reduced functional capacity, with function improving once neovascularization occurs (Anderson et al., 1989; Korsgren et al., 1999). There is a correlation between the number of islet equivalents (IE) transplanted per kg (IE/kg) (Sutherland et al., 2008), but there is considerable overlap in functional outcome (Blondet et al., 2007). A few (~7%) IAT recipients of <2500 IE/kg become insulin-independent while about a third with >5000 IE/kg do not (Sutherland et al., 2008). Most likely this relates to differences in viability between different islet preparations: a low islet yield with a high percentage of viable islets will out-perform a high islet yield with a low percentage of viable islets, a hypothesis supported by the studies by Papas et al. (2010) showing the best predictor of islet function in IAT recipients was the in vitro oxygen consumption rate prior to implantation (Papas et al., 2010).

To prevent intraportal clotting from the tissue thromboplastin (present in the islet preparation) (Mehigan et al., 1980), the authors have administered heparin since their first cases in the 1970s (Najarian et al., 1979; Wahoff et al., 1995a). Nearly all of the reports of complications related to portal infusion of islets (Mehigan et al., 1980; Memsic et al., 1984; Toledo-Pereyra et al., 1984; Walsh et al., 1982), were published before the standardized semi-automated pancreas dispersion techniques and before the routine use of heparinization at all centers. A recent analysis of the authors' data indicates that the incidence of complications of IAT is low if less than 0.25 ml tissue/kg is infused (Wilhelm et al., 2011). If the volume is higher, consideration should be given to volume reduction even though some islets are lost, or to simply transplant less than the full unpurified islet mass. There is some risk of heparinization in patients who have heparin antibodies, with one case of heparin induced thrombocytopenia reported after TP-IAT (Rastellini et al., 2006).

In regard to technical aspects of intraportal islet infusion, the most simple technique is to wait for the islets after the enteric and biliary reconstruction has been done following TP and to infuse the islets directly into the portal vein or a tributary and then close the patient (Blondet et al., 2007). However, techniques also exist for intraportal embolizaiont of islet so the liver after abdominal closure has been obtained. The techniques include emoblization to a temporarily exteriorized omental vein (Nath et al., 2004); via a recanalized umbilical vein (Pollard et al., 2011) or percutaneous transhepatic access to the portal vein for infusion of the islets (Morgan et al., 2011). The latter approach frees up surgeons and an operating room for other procedures sooner than if the islets are infused in the operating room and thus is thought to be cost-effective at least at one center (Morgan et al., 2011), but the expense incurred by using interventional radiology must also be considered as well as the fact that the abdomen cannot be inspected for bleeding after the heparinization and increased portal pressure that ensue by lieu of the infusion (Blondet et al., 2007).

In islet allograft recipients, one study by Doppler ultrasound showed a 4% incidence of radiologically detected but clinically insignificant portal vein thrombosis (Casey et al., 2002). The risk factors for portal vein thrombosis in islet allograft recipients has been delineated and primarily relates to tissue volume and degree of anticoagulation in the early post-infusion period (Kawahara et al., 2011). In the authors' IAT series, portal vein thrombosis occasionally is detected on ultrasound, but not as a clinical entity (Sutherland et al., 2011b). The authors always administer heparin before islet infusion and usually continue the infusion for a few days if the closing portal pressures are high. Liver function tests typically show a transient rise in serum enzyme levels during the early postoperative period (Gores et al., 1992), with no implication for future hepatic dysfunction. Imaging studies of the liver after IAT often do show changes, such as echogenic nodularity, but such changes do not appear to be associated with any clinical problems and thus are benign (Ong et al., 2008).

8. Intra- and post-operative considerations

The authors maintain euglycemia by an insulin drip during and after the pancreatectomy and IAT (Manciu et al., 1999) . Animal studies have shown a decrease in islet engraftment with hyperglycemia; furthermore, glucose toxicity may cause dysfunction and structural lesions in the transplanted islets (Bellin et al., 2009; Clark et al., 1982; Dohan & Lukens ,1947; Korsgren et al., 1989; Makhlouf et al., 2003). The authors promote islet engraftment by an exogenous insulin drip to maintain euglycemia, minimizing insulin secretory demand from the freshly infused islets. A transition to subcutaneous insulin is made when the patient begins to eat or is on a tube-feeding regimen if eating is delayed, with the dose again adjusted to maintain euglycemia; insulin gradually is withdrawn in patients who can achieve euglycemia without it, but this is rarely done before 6 months.

9. Expanding application

IATs have been done after pancreatic resection for focal benign pancreatic processes, including pancreatic pseudocysts (Clayton et al., 2003) cystic neoplasms such as intrapapillary mucinous neoplasms IPMN (Berney et al. 2004; Lee et al., 2005), insulinomas (Berney T et al., 2004; Oberholzer et al. 2003) neuroendocrine and other tumors (Berney T et al., 2004; Ris; 2011). In a series of 14 patients in Seoul, Korea with a mixture of benign tumors, including IPMN (Jung et al., 2009), pathologic evaluation was completed in each before the IAT to confirm that the lesions were benign.

In the UMN series, IATs have been done at the time of distal pancreatectomy for benign cystic tumors in 5 patients (Blondet et al., 2007; Braganza et al., 2011). In these cases the authors are uncertain how well the intrahepatic islets are functioning, because those in the native pancreatic remnant also are functioning.

In the Seoul series mentioned above (Jung et al., 2009), however, the investigators did a formal comparison of 14 patients who had partial pancreatectomy (PP) with an IAT and 6 who had PP without an IAT. Glucose tolerance was abruptly impaired in both groups immediately after surgery, including reduced indices of insulin secretion, but beginning at 6 months and persisting at 24 months, the PP-IAT group had statistically better insulin secretion and glucose tolerance than the PP-alone group. Thus, even with a PP there is a metabolic advantage to doing an IAT; and this would especially be the case if a completion pancreatectomy has to be done later for any reason. The lessons from the Korean experience can be extended to the CP group where a partial pancreatctomy before a completion pancreatectomy is quite common (usually a Whipple, but sometimes a distal).

An IAT also has been reported in a patient with pancreatic adenocarcinoma who had an extended Whipple operation complicated by an anastomotic leak at the pancreaticojejunostomy (Forster et al., 2004). . The leak was treated by an urgent completion pancreatectomy with an IAT. The portion of the pancreas used for islet isolation had margins free of tumor. The patient remained C-peptide positive until death from metastases 2.5 years later, but there was no tumor in the liver.

The risk of doing an IAT when a completion pancreatectomy is done because of a technical complication of a Whipple procedure cannot be calculated from one case, but conceptually the procedure is valid, because the judgment must be that the distal pancreas was tumor-free by leaving it in (otherwise a Whipple operation would not have been done). A case also could be made for doing a TP-IAT, even in situations where a Whipple would otherwise suffice, but where a TP would be safer by avoiding an enteric anastomosis to a soft pancreas that has a higher than average leakage or breakdown probability These cases are anecdotal and there is at this time no technique to assure that isolated islets are not contaminated by tumor. However, at least for hereditary CP with gene mutations associated with risk for pancreatic cancer, there are no reports yet of cancer arising in the liver after TP-IAT, including those done more than 20 years ago (Blondet et al., 2007).

A case can be made for doing a TP-IAT in patients with hereditary chronic pancreatitis in whom pain is not an issue (for example, "burned out") but has reached the age (>35 years) where the risk of pancreatic cancer associated with the gene mutations is significant and it increases with age (Farrow & Evers, 2002; Whitcomb, 2004; Whitcomb & Pogue-Geile, 2002).

On another note, the authors' TP-IAT series includes a few CP patients whose IATs were done after only a distal pancreatectomy, with the head remaining (Sutherland et al., 2011b). For those in whom a completion pancreatectomy was done later, insulin-independence was preserved, indicating good engraftment at the initial IAT (Blondet et al., 2007).

Transplants of islets isolated from pancreas allografts excised for technical problems or allograft pancreatitis (islet auto-allografts) also have been performed, with one case published by the authors (Leone et al., 1998) . This patient remained insulin-independent for more than 1 year while on immunosuppression, but ultimately needed exogenous insulin from decline or loss of islet function for immunologic or non-immunologic reasons. The other islet auto-allografts had limited duration of function (Blondet et al., 2007).

10. Islet autotransplantation in children

CP is less common in children than in adults, but should be treated with the same aim: to relieve pain, eliminate the need for narcotics, and preserve ß-cell mass (Schmulewitz, 2011). The first known case of TP-IAT in a child was done at the University of Minnesota in 1989 and was reported in detail by the authors 7 years later with islet function maintained, though the patient was not insulin-independent (Wahoff et al., 1996). The authors have done TP-IAT in more than 40 children since the initial report (Bellin & Sutherland, 2010). Although the experience with TPIAT in children is less extensive than in adults, the data suggests this procedure is particularly successful in the youngest patients with insulin-independence rates of over 50% and the younger the patient the more likely insulin-independence is achieved (Bellin et al., 2008a; Bellin & Sutherland, 2010). Most of the ones that do require insulin retain some beta cell function as manifested by C-peptide positivity and thus are stable. In the historical series, more than three-quarters of the children had islet function after TP-IAT (Bellin et al., 2008a) Brittle diabetes is very rare after TP-IAT unless virtually no islets are obtained because of delaying the TP until nearly all the islets are destroyed by the disease process (Bellin & Sutherland, 2010; Kobayashi et al., 2010)

Most important is the effect of TP-IAT on the CP pain syndrome. Sixty to seventy percent of children completely discontinue narcotic pain medications, while the majority of the remaining patients require only intermittent or low dose narcotics for pain control (Bellin et al., 2008a; Bellin et al., 2011b). Complete discontinuation of narcotics is more frequent in preadolescent patients (younger than 13 years of age) (Bellin et al., 2008a). Over 90% of all children report no pain or significant improvement in pain compared to before surgery (Bellin et al., 2008a). Health-related quality of life, as measured by the Medical Outcomes Study (MOS) Short-Form 36 (SF-36) is nearly two standard deviations below the population at baseline but normalizes on average by 1 year postoperatively (Bellin et al., 2011b).

The islet auto-transplant procedure is the same in children as that performed in adults. Including the cases done outside the University Of Minnesota, IATs have been performed in at least 50 children (not all published) with the majority of islet grafts infused intraportally (Bellin et al., 2008a; Bellin et al., 2011b; Sutherland et al., 2011a). There is one case report of intramuscular autoislet transplant in a 7 year old child; this patient had documented graft function and good metabolic control for over 2 years post-IAT but did not achieve insulin independence (Rafael et al., 2008). In children undergoing intraportal IAT, 40-50% of patients achieve insulin independence in the first 1 year after IAT, with the highest rate of insulin independence in preadolescent children (Bellin & Sutherland, 2010). In addition to young age, higher islet mass transplanted and lack of prior distal resection and/or lateral pancreatico-jejunostomy are important prognostic factors for insulin independence (Bellin et al., 2008a; Bellin et al., 2011b). More extensive fibrosis and longer duration of disease have been associated with lower islet yields and hence higher risk of insulin dependence in children (Kobayashi et al., 2010). As in adults, baseline glucose, C-peptide (fasting and stimulated), and hemoglobin A1c are measured before surgery. Lower hemoglobin A1c, lower fasting blood glucose, and higher stimulated C-peptide levels are associated with higher islet yields but do not predict the islet count prior to pancreatectomy for any individual patient (Bellin et al., 2010a)

Most important of all is the dramatic improvement in quality of life that can be documented in children undergoing TP-IAT for CP, both retrospectively (Bellin et al., 2008a) and in a recent prospective study at the University Of Minnesota (Bellin et al., 2011b). In the prospective study, nineteen consecutive children (aged 5–18 years) undergoing TP/IAT from December 2006 to December 2009 at the University of Minnesota completed the Medical Outcomes Study 36-item Short Form (SF-36) health questionnaire before and after surgery. Before TP/IAT, the children had below average health-related quality of life, based on data from the Medical Outcomes Study SF-36; they had a mean physical component summary (PCS) score of 30 and mental component summary (MCS) score of 34 (2 and 1.5 standard deviations, respectively, below the mean for the US population). By 1 year after surgery, PCS and MCS scores significantly improved to 50 and 46, respectively Mean scores improved for all 8 component subscales. More than 60% of IAT recipients were insulin independent or required minimal insulin. Patients with prior surgical drainage procedures (Puestow) had significantly lower yields of islets and greater incidence of insulin dependence

Although the number of patients is relatively small, this study (Bellin et al., 2011b) shows that the physical and emotional components that define quality of life significantly improve after TP/IAT in subsets of pediatric patients with CP. Children who have had surgical drainage procedures prior to TP-IAT are disadvantaged in regard to islet yield and none yet have had sustained insulin independence,; however even in this subset some had islet function as manifested by C-peptide positivity or need for only once daily long acting insulin. Children should not be allowed to suffer the pain of CP when it can be relieved by TP and beta cell function preserved by IAT, and quality of life is restored in nearly all cases.

11. Literature review

The largest series published to date on patients undergoing pancreatectomy and IAT have come from the University of Minnesota (Farney et al., 1991; Gores et al., 1992; Gruessner et al., 2004; Jie et al., 2005; Najarian et al., 1979; Najarian et al., 1980; Sutherland et al., 1978; Sutherland et al., 1980a; Sutherland et al., 2004a; Sutherland et al., 2009a; Sutherland et al., 2009b; Sutherland et al., 2011b; Wahoff et al., 1995a) (>400), the University of Cincinnati (Ahmad et al., 2005; Rodriguez et al., 2003; Sutton et al., 2010) (>100), the University of Leicester (Clayton et al., 2003;; Garcea et al., 2009; White SA et al., 1998; White SA et al., 2001; Webb et al., 2008) (>50 cases), but there are many center that are building their series (Argo et al., 2008; Berney T et al., 2000; Desai et al., 2011; Dixon et al., 2008; Jahansouz et al., 2011; Takita et al., 2010; Takita et al., 2011b; Valente et al., 1986) The reports from these centers largely focus on metabolic outcomes, QOL, and pain reduction., but there are many publications on specialized aspects of TP-IAT as have been referenced in this chapter.

11.1 Insulin independence

The ability to achieve insulin independence after IATs appears to correlate directly with the islet equivalents (IEs) infused. IEs serve as an indirect measurement of β-cell mass, but there is much overlap, in that a small percentage of patients receiving less than 2000 IE/kg will become insulin-independent, while some receiving more than 5000 IE/kg will not (Ahmad et al., 2005; Bellin et al., 2009; Blondet et al., 2007; Dong et al., 2011; Jie et al., 2005; Sutherland et al., 2008; Sutherland et al., 2009a; Takita et al., 2011a). The Leicester group finds very little correlation of insulin-independence with islet yield (Webb et al., 2008). The authors have shown that islet yields are poorest in patients who have prior pancreatic resections (distal pancreatectomies or surgical drainage procedures such as the Puestow procedure) (Blondet et al., 2007; Gruessner et al., 2004; Sutherland et al., 2011b; Wahoff et al.,1995c). In addition, fewer islets are recovered as histopathologic changes of CP increase in severity (Gruessner et al., 2004; Kobayashi et al., 2010; Kobayashi et al., 2011; Wahoff et al., 1995a).

The timing of the procedure has a direct impact on islet yield. Maximal islet yield and insulin independence may be attained more easily if the IAT is performed earlier in the disease course, (Ahmad et al., 2006; Balamurugan et al., 2011a; Bellin et al., 2010a; Kobayashi et al., 2011; Rodriguez et al., 2003; Sutherland et al., 2011; Takita et al., 2010).

In regard to durability of insulin independence when it is achieved after TP-IAT, it is much more durable than in islet allografts, even though the number of islets transplanted is less than for islet allografts (Sutherland et al., 2008). In a retrospective analysis of the first 173 patients to undergo TP-IAT at the University of Minnesota (20 year follow-up on the longest), the incidence of graft function and insulin-independence and decline over time once achieved was calculated and compared to the same calculations made for islet allografts in the Collaborative Islet Transplant Registry (CITR) (Figure 3).

Islet allografts are currently associated with a high rate of early insulin independence, but after 1 year insulin-independence rates have declined relatively rapidly in the CITR analyses overall (CITR; 2009) and at most (Jahansouz et al., 2011) but, more recently, not all (Bellin et al., 2008b) institutions,. The 2008 analysis of islet auto-transplants (IATs) done at the University Of Minnesota over a 30 year period in those who achieved function showed to be relatively durable compared to the islet allografts, despite a lower beta-cell mass (Bellin et al., 2008b). IAT function (full/partial combined) and insulin independence correlated with islet yield. Overall only 65% functioned within the first year, and only 32% were insulin independent, but of IATs that functioned initially, 85% remained so 2-years later, in contrast to 66% of allografts Of IAT recipients who became insulin independent, 74%remained so 2-years later versus 45%of initially insulin-independent allograft recipients. Of IATs that functioned or induced insulin independence, the rates at 5 years were 69% and 47%, respectively. Thus, islet function is more resilient in autografts than allografts. Indeed, in this analysis, the 5-year insulin-independence persistence rate for IATs was similar to the 2-year rate for allografts. Several factors unique to allocases are likely responsible for the differences, including donor brain death, longer cold ischemia time, diabetogenic immunosuppression, and auto- and alloimmunity. IAT outcomes provide a minimum theoretical standard to work

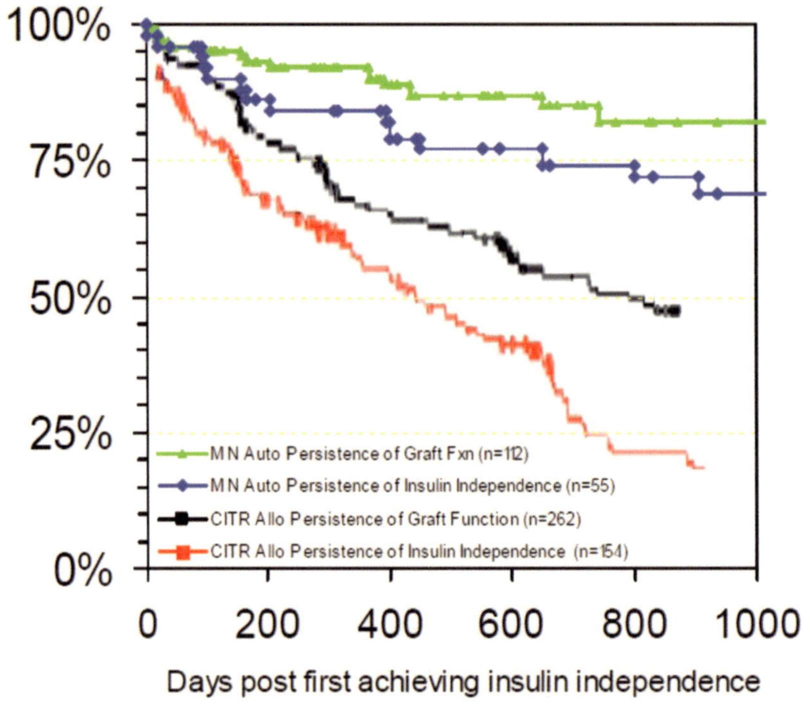

Fig. 3. Rates of loss of islet graft function or insulin independence (II) in University Of Minnesota 1977 to 2007 adult TP recipients of islet AUTO-transplants who achieved islet function or II versus in 1999-2006 type 1 diabetic recipients of islet ALLO-transplants who likewise achieved islet function or II as reported to the Collaborative Islet Transplant Registry (CITR) (Reproduced from Sutherland et al., 2008; with Copyright ©, Lippincott Williams & Wilkins, Inc.)

toward in allotransplantation. However, not all islet autografts that initially function continue to do so, and beta cell mass is important, the more the islets, the more durable the function, particularly in adults. Preadolescent children are a special group where even a low islet mass can function long term, and possibly the mass expands in young children (Bellin & Sutherland, 2010).

11.1.1 University of Minnesota series

As referenced above, the University Of Minnesota has published extensively on their series of TP-IAT cases, numbering more than 400 between 1977 and 2011 (Fig 4). In a comprehensive 1995 report (Wahoff et al., 1995a), of the first 50 cases, significant pain relief occurred in >80%. Over half had a period of insulin-independence and a third maintained insulin independence for the 2 to 10 years they had been followed. If over 300,000 islets were transplanted, three-quarters maintained insulin independence by the protocol in place at the time (which did not include adding insulin for perturbations in metabolism as we do now). A major point of this paper (Wahoff et al., 1995a) was that the lowest islet yields were in patients who had a prior Puestow procedure, with only an 18% rate of insulin independence in this group, in contrast to 71% in patients without a prior resection or drainage procedure.

In a later update of the UMN series, at a time when the authors were much more likely to treat even mild hyperglycemia, and nearly all patients underwent a TP, insulin independence was achieved in only 16% of patients with prior resections versus 40% in those without prior resections (Gruessner et al., 2004) . A prior Whipple operation had less effect on the islet yield than a distal pancreatectomy (Sutherland et al., 2004a) .

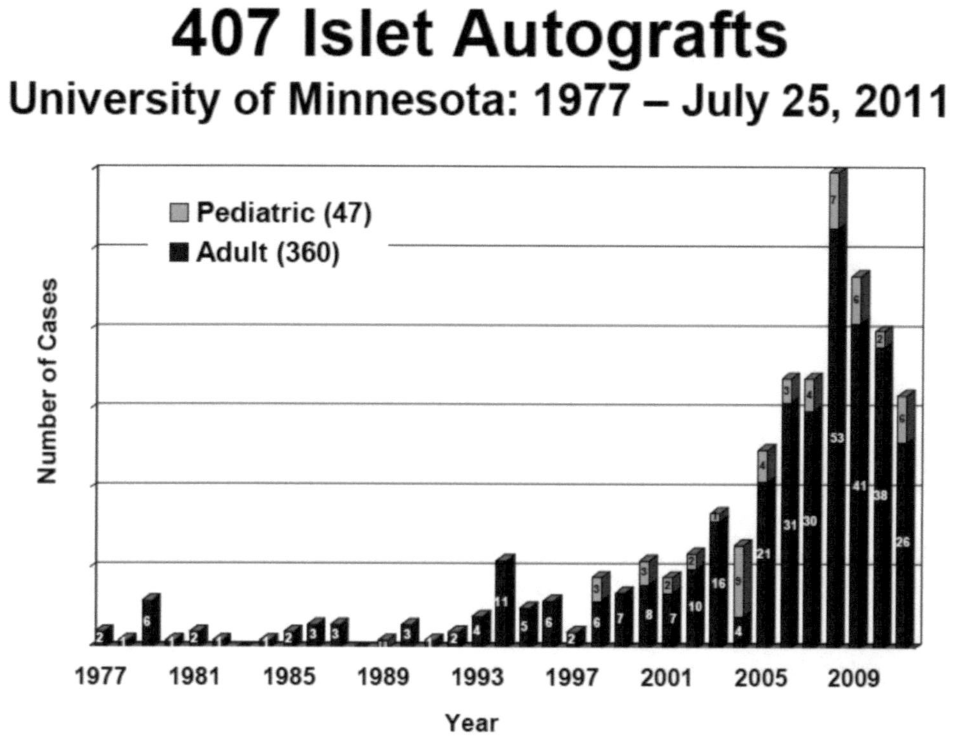

Fig. 4. Islet autograft experience at the University of Minnesota by year, in 407 patients (360 adults, 47 children <18 years old) from February 1977 to July 2011.

The outcomes in the University of Minnesota series were again updated in 2005 when it included 136 patients 971% female) undergoing IAT from 1977 through 2004 (Jie et al., 2005). Further details on this cohort were added in 2007 (Blondet et al., 2007). Patient age ranged from 5 to 70 years (mean 36 years); duration of disease ranged from 1 to 30 years (mean 5.9 years). The etiology of CP was idiopathic in 43%, alcohol in 15%, divisum in 13%, familial in 11%, biliary in 10% and other in 7% of the patients. Most (93%) had had previous operations (cholecystectomy in 42%), 33% directly on the pancreas including duct drainage in 13%, Whipple procedure in 7%, distal pancreatectomy in 9% and combined drainage and resection in 4%. .

A TP or completion pancreatectomy was done in 77% and a near total (duodenal sparing) in 15%, while 10 had a distal pancreatectomy only (some later had a completion pancreatectomy). This analysis (Jie et al.; 2005) confirmed that a prior Puestow procedure was associated with low islet yields (mean of 1531 IE/kg) as compared to no previous direct surgery on the pancreas (mean of 3996 IE/kg). Prior resection was associate with a slightly lower yield (3687 IE/kg), but the difference was much more striking after a distal pancreatectomy than a Whipple operation. Again, there was a correlation between islet yield and insulin independence. Of patients receiving >2000 IEQ/kg, nearly three-quarters had at least a period off insulin (Jie et al., 2005). Of those completely dependent on insulin, the mean IE/kg transplanted was 1239, while in those in whom it was intermittent it was 3064; in those who maintained insulin-independence it was 5118/kg. About a third of patients fall into each category (Blondet et al., 2007).

Most important was formal patient self-assessment of quality of life after TP-IAT as the University Of Minnesota program progressed (Carlson et al., 2007). Of 90 patients transplanted between 1996 and 2005 with >1 year follow-up in all, 83% reported good to excellent outcome and less than 5% considered their outcomes poor [Figure 5]. This retrospective survey has since been followed by prospective studies of quality of life in both children and adults in the Minnesota series.

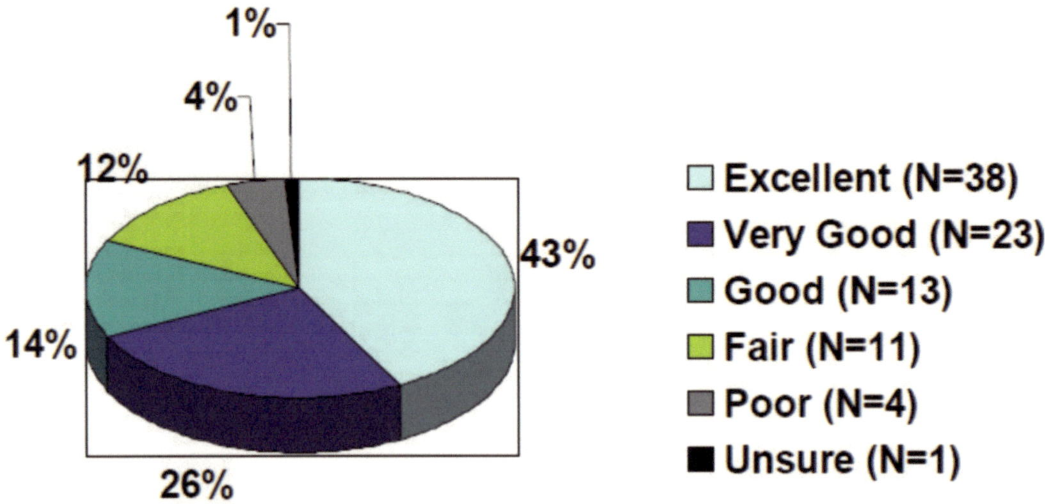

Fig. 5. Patient subjective perception of their outcome post-TP-IAT (1-10 years follow-up) , for 1996-2005 adult cases at University of Minnesota (data from Carlson et al 2007).

Patient survival and durability of IAT graft function (either insulin-independent or on once daily insulin only and C-peptide positive) and insulin-independence in the Minnesota TP-IAT series for 1977-2007 cases (Figure 6) was detailed in a 2008 publication (Sutherland et al., 2008). Patient survival at 1 year was 95% and more than three-quarters were alive at 10 years. More than two thirds had partial or full function of the IAT, with a third achieving insulin independence. At 20 years more than half who exhibited IAT function initially still had function, so overall more than one-third of the original cohort had functioning islets for two decades in this series that includes the earliest cases. Half of those who were insulin independent initially were still so at 5 years; none were insulin-independent at 20 years but at least partial function was maintained for at least this length.(Figure 6). The durability of IAT function (Figure 7) and of insulin-independence (Figure 8) in those who did initially achieve partial or full function, correlated with the number of islets transplanted. For those receiving >5000 IE/kg, more than three quarters still had function (full and partial combined) 5 years later, while it was slightly less than half for those who received <2500 IE/kg (Figure 7). Similarly, of those who achieved insulin independence, nearly three-quarters of those who received >5000 IE/kg were still insulin-independent 5 years later, while it was less than a third for those who received <2500 IE/kg (Figure 8).

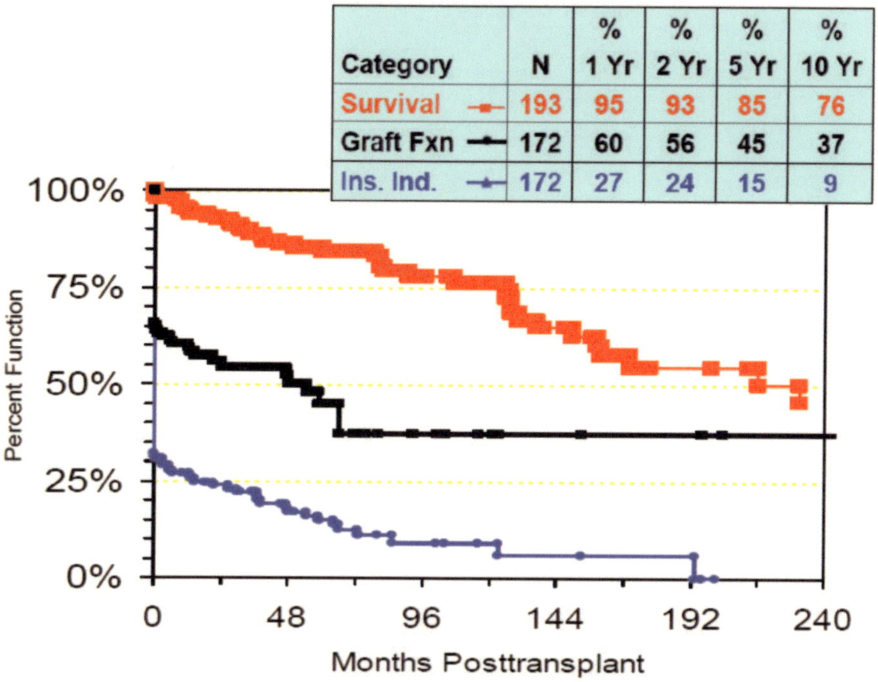

Fig. 6. Actuarial patient survival rates, IAT graft function rates(full-partial combined) and insulin-independence rates from time of transplant for adult Patients undergoing TP-IAT at University Of Minnesota from 1977 to 2007 (data from Sutherland et al, 2008)

Since many modifications in islet isolation, surgical technique and patient selection have occurred over the decades since the first TP-IAT case, the outcomes at the University Of Minnesota in the modern era alone have been the subject of recent analyses of pain relief and quality of life (Sutherland et al., 2009a) and metabolic outcome (Sutherland et al., 2009b). Of 67 adult patients undergoing TP-IAT for CP between January, 2006 and February 2008 (Sutherland et al., 2009a), all had had attempts at pain relief by prior endoscopic duct drainage (EDD) procedures. In all the pain had persisted in spite of the EDD. EDD is a minimally invasive approach that should almost always be tried before major surgery for CP, but in these 67 patients the pain had persisted in spite of the EDD.

The patients were assessed by written surveys and clinic interviews and metabolic testing in 2009, with more than 1 year of follow-up (16-44 months) in all (Sutherland et al., 2009a). Mean age was 36 years and 72% were female. Etiology of CP was unknown in 40%); from pancreas divisums in 14%; genetic in 14%; associated with Sphincter of Oddi dysfunction (SOD) in 12%; with alcohol use in 9%; and other in 11%. Patients were surveyed for outcomes with a median follow-up of 1.7yrs Actual survival at 1 year was 98.5%; actuarial survival at 2 years was 95.5%. The collective number of EDD procedures prior to surgery was 264 (mean of

IEQ/kg	N	1 Yr fx	5 Yr fx
> 5,000	32	97%	78%
2,501–5,000	56	92%	74%
< 2,500	24	88%	49%

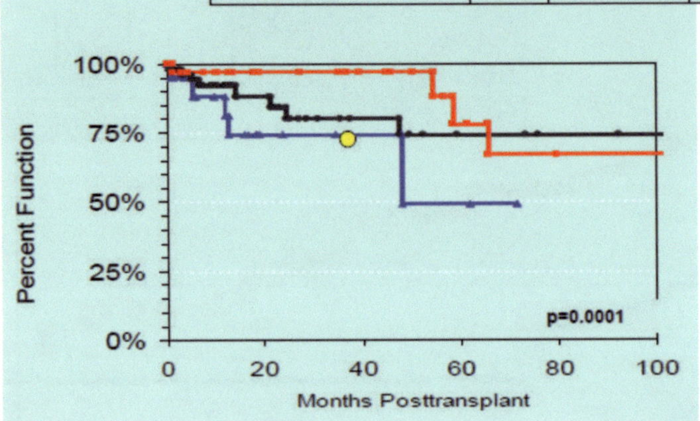

Fig. 7. Actuarial duration of islet graft function (full-partial combined) according to islet yield in adult patients who achieved function after TP-IAT at University Of Minnesota from 1977 to 2007 (data from Sutherland et al, 2008).

IEQ/kg	N	1 Yr fx	5 Yr fx
> 5,000	23	100%	71%
2,501–5,000	24	77%	46%
< 2,500	8	60%	30%

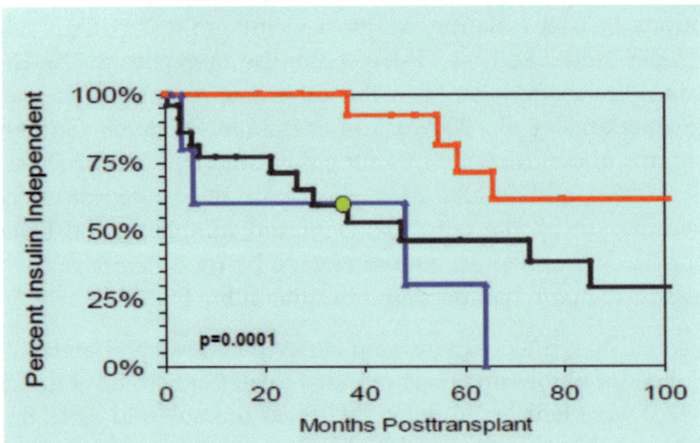

Fig. 8. Actuarial duration of insulin independence according to islet yield in adult patients who achieved insulin-independence after TP-IAT at University Of Minnesota from 1977 to 2007 (data from Sutherland et al, 2008).

4.1/patient; max ~60). Ten patients (15%) had had a partial pancreatectomy elsewhere before a total (completion) pancreatectomy-IAT at the University Of Minnesota, and did not have EDD in the interval.

Patients were assessed at follow-up for pain, narcotic use, quality of life (QOL) and IAT function: full if insulin-independent; partial if euglycemic on once daily long-acting insulin; failed if on a basal-bolus insulin regime). Function was correlated with islet (IE) yield.

Yield was:

<2500 IE/kg in 22 (34%);
2501-5000 IE/kg in 30 (46%);
>5000 IE/kg in 13 (20%).

IAT function was:

Full in 21 (32 %);
partial in 28 (43 %);
failed in 16 (25 %).

IAT function was a combined

full-partial in:100% with >5000 IE/kg;
83% with 2501-5000 IE/kg;
and 59% with <2500 IE/kg (p<.0011).

Perception of health was:

good-excellent in 75 %;
fair in14 %;
poor in 11 %.

Pain was:

better in 85 %(absent in 39 %);
the same in 13 %;
worse in 2 %.

97 % were on narcotics before the TP-IAT; 51 % were on at the time of the post-surgery survey (85% of these were on a wean schedule).

Of those who required insulin, 98% preferred diabetes to the former pain.

Patients rated quality of life (QOL) after TP-IAT as:

excellent-good in 60 %;
fair in 30 %;
poor in 10 %.

QOL change from before to after TP-IAT:

improved in 80 %;
was the same in 15 %;
was worse in 5 %.

Asked would they do the TP-IAT again, 98% said yes.

In these modern era studies (Braganza et al., 2011; Casadei et al., 2010a) in patients with pain after EDD for CP, TP-IAT gave relief in most, preserved meaningful insulin secretion in three-fourths, and improved QOL in four-fifths. Nearly all would do the TP-IAT again, but that fact that not all would indicates an effort is needed to identify in advance patients who will not be made better. Right now that is difficult to do, so to help the many who can be helped, a few will have to be resigned to failure but the percentage is low, and in this study improvement in quality of life was often strikingly dramatic.

The latest analysis of the Minnesota IAT series of IAT includes >400 cases as of mid-2011 (Sutherland et al., 2011b), more than half of them since 2006 (Fig. 3). The results are briefly summarized here.

The etiology of CP in the entire series is currently classified as idiopathic in 44%; sphincter of Oddi dysfunction or biliary in 16%; genetic-in 15%; divisum in 2%; alcohol in only 8%; other in 5%). At least 1 yr follow-up outcomes were available in 313 patients (278 adults, mean age 35.6 yrs,; and 35 children); 74% were female; prior-surgeries had been done in 25%--Peustow- y in 7%, resection in 18%) done before June 2009. Islet-function was considered full for patients insulin-independent; partial if euglycemic on once-daily-insulin; and failed if on a standard-diabetic-regimen even if C-peptide-positive. The SF-36-survey (Quality-of-Life (QOL)) was retrospectively completed by 101 patients done before Sep/2006 and prospectively before and after TP-IAT in 201 patients thereafter.

The results showed actuarial-patient-survival post-TP-IAT was 96% in adults and 98% in children (1-year) and; 89% and 98% (5-years). Overall, IAT-function was achieved in 70% (insulin-independence in 28%); 69% (25%) in adults, 78% (52%) in children. Prior-surgery lowered islet-yield (2712vs4077/kg,p=.003). Islet yield [<2500/kg (38%); 2501-5000/kg (34%); >5000/kg (28%)] correlated with glucose control: full-partial rates at 1-year: 26, 79 and 82%, respectively; insulin-independence rates:5, 41 and 65%. All adults retrospectively (1977-2006) surveyed had pain before TP-IAT and 95% were on daily-narcotics. Afterwards, 94% had pain-improvement and 49% ceased-narcotics. 85% of adults stated QOL improved; 8% stated it was same; 5% said it was worse. All children were on narcotics before, 39% at follow-up; pain improved in 94%; 67% became pain-free. In the prospective-QOL-study-since-2006, there was improvement after TP-IAT in all 8 SF-36-subscale-scores (p<0.001) with the greatest effect on bodily-pain, as was previously reported in another publication (Bellin et al., 2011c).

In this prospective study of health related quality of life (HRQoL) of patients transplanted since September 2006 (mean age 37, 77% female), prior to surgery, mean Physical Component Score (PCS) was 27 and Mental Component Score (MCS) was 32 (standardized normal=50, SD=10). Both PCS and MCS significantly improved after surgery. At 1 and 2 years, mean PCS scores were 37 and 42 respectively and MCS scores were 42 and 46. Change in PCS from baseline to 1y was greater for children than adults (+15 v. +10). All 8 subscale scores significantly improved over time), with the greatest effect on bodily pain. Children demonstrated more rapid improvement, particularly for bodily pain and role physical.

This prospective study showed meaningful improvement in HRQoL after TPIAT. Although the greatest improvement was in bodily pain, other dimensions of physical, social, and emotional health improved.

This large series, as well as those of others cited above and below, shows definitively that TP can ameliorate pain and improve QOL in patients with otherwise refractory CP, , even if narcotic-withdrawal is delayed or incomplete because of prior long-term use. IAT preserves substantial islet-function in >2/3 of patients with insulin-independence occurring in a quarter of adults and half the children.

11.1.2 Cincinnati series

The Cincinnati series of TP-IAT cases (Ahmad et al., 2005; Ahmad et al., 2006; Sutton et al., 2010) is the second largest in the literature with their latest report including 118 cases (Sutton et al., 2010). The early reports from this group (Ahmad et al., 2005; Ahmad et al., 2006) showed a 40% rate of insulin independence after TP/IAT, with a mean follow-up of 18 months. Factors that correlated with postoperative insulin independence included the patient's weight, body mass index (BMI), and gender (Rodriguez Rilo et al., 2003). Patients who had a BMI greater than 28 had a higher chance of insulin dependence (Rodriguez Rilo et al., 2003). Reduction to ideal body weight to minimize insulin resistance may maximize the chance for insulin independence after TP-IAT. Insulin-independent patients had lower mean insulin requirements during the first 24 hours after transplant, possibly relating to the detrimental effect of hyperglycemia on islet function (Ahmad et al., 2006). Of their first 54 CP patients who underwent a TP-IAT ,about two thirds had discontinued narcotics at the time of the report and two-thirds had full or partial islet function, (Ahmad et al., 2006). The most recent report from Cincinnati on their TP-IAT series focuses on 16 patients (out of 118, or 14%) with genetic mutations associated with CP (Sutton et al., 2010)[. At a mean follow-up of 22 months, 69% of patients had good islet function and 25% were insulin-independent. All were on narcotics before TP-IAT while only 37% were at follow-up and at lower doses.. An SF-36 survey and pain questionnaire in this cohort demonstrated significant improvement in quality of life and reduction or elimination of pain following TP-IAT for genetically linked pancreatitis. The Cincinnati experience shows that patients with painful hereditary pancreatitis respond well to TP-IAT and should be considered for early intervention in the course of their disease.

11.1.3 Leicester series

The Leicester series of TP-IAT for CP is the third largest in the literature with more than 50 cases since 1996 (Clayton et al., 2003; Garcea et al., 2009; Webb et al., 2008; Ong et al., 2008). Interestingly, early reports from Leicester did not show a correlation between islet yield and insulin independence (Clayton et al., 2003), in contrast to the Minnesota series (Blondet et al., 2007; Sutherland et al., 2009b; Wahoff et al., 1995a). The results may relate to the cause of the CP (mostly alcohol) and possibly to patient compliance issues (Clayton et al., 2003).

The two most recent publications of the Leicester TP-IAT series for CP focus on metabolic outcomes (Webb et al., 2008) and on pain and narcotic reduction or elimination (Garcea et al., 2009), with a comparison in the latter paper to patients with CP who underwent only a TP. In the paper assessing long term IAT graft function in 46 IAT recipients (followup 2-63 months, median 16.5 months), all (100%) were C-peptide function and therefore had functioning islets. Twelve achieved insulin-independence for 2-63 months (median 16.5 months) and 5 remain insulin-independent. Over time insulin requirement tended to increase as did glycohemoglobin levels but all the recipients remained C-peptide positive for up to 10 years (maximum follow-up). They also assessed renal function over time and it was stable in all suggesting diabetic nephropathy did not occur to any significant degree. The main point of the paper was that even though a decline in IAT function over time could be detected, total loss of function did not occur and protection against diabetic complications was likely (Webb et al., 2008).

In the other recent paper from Leicester (Garcea et al., 2009) the focus was on a comparison of 85 patients who underwent TP for CP, 50 with and 35 without an IAT. In the entire series, 90% of patients were on narcotics at the time of surgery; it fell to 40% by one year and 16% by 5 years. At 5 years insulin requirements were significantly lower in the IAT group, median of 16 units per 24 hours vs. 40 units in the TP alone group and 5 patients in the IAT group were insulin-independent.

The Leicester series complements those of other centers, as described above in the previous sections, in showing the effectiveness of TP in reducing or eliminating the pain of CP and in documenting the metabolic benefit of adding an IAT to the procedure.

11.2 Comments

Insulin independence is only partially the goal of an IAT, because preserving any β-cell mass is beneficial (Pezzilli, 2006; Robertson, 2010a). Indeed, islet allograft recipients who remain insulin dependent but have β-cell function and are C-peptide positive are metabolically more stable and less prone to hypoglycemic unawareness than those who have no β-cell function (Jahansouz et al., 2011; Paty et al., 2006; Robertson, 2010b; Ryan et al., 2002; Ryan et al., 2005). Furthermore, the risk of secondary complications is less in diabetics who receive or are C-peptide-positive (Jahansouz et al., 2011; Johansson et al., 2000; Kamiya et al., 2004). By extrapolation, IAT recipients who are C-peptide-positive, even with an insulin requirement, have a metabolic advantage (Dong et al., 2011). Although only about one-third or less of IAT recipients in the various series are insulin-independent long-term; another third have enough islets to achieve near-normoglycemia with exogenous insulin, usually with one injection daily of the long-acting variety (Bellin et al., 2009; Jie et al., 2005; Sutherland et al., 2009b; Sutherland et al., 2011b), and even those who are on basal-bolus insulin regimens are usually C-peptide positive in the modern era (Sutherland et al., 2011b; Webb et al., 2008).

Although about one third of IAT recipients in the various series require a basal-bolus insulin regimen because of low viable islet yield (Jie et al., 2005; Sutherland et al., 2004a; Sutherland et al., 2011b), as long as pain is relieved or improved, the operation is considered a success. One should only do a TP-IAT in patients who are fully informed about the risk of becoming diabetic, and who accept this risk in exchange for reasonable chances at both pain reduction and narcotic withdrawal. Some patients who became fully diabetic after TP-IAT because of inadequate viable islet yield, and who were particularly labile, have gone on to have a pancreas (allograft) transplant, and thus achieved insulin independence (Gruessner et al., 2004; Gruessner et al., 2008), but at the expense of needing immunosuppression (Sutherland et al., 2001).. An islet allograft also could be done in this situation (Sakata et al., 2008), but an enteric-drained pancreas transplant is more attractive, because exocrine deficiency also can be corrected (Gruessner et al., 2004; Gruessner et al., 2008).

12. Long-term metabolic outcomes

One long-term study of metabolic outcomes in six TP-IAT recipients from the authors' center reported that diabetes mellitus was prevented for up to 13 (now 20) years (mean follow-up at study, 6.2 plus or minus 1.7 years) (Robertson et al., 2001). Normal fasting plasma glucose, intravenous glucose disappearance rate (κG), hemoglobin A_{1c}, insulin responses to intravenous glucose and arginine, and insulin secretory reserve were maintained, but insulin responses tended to decrease over time. The intravenous glucose disappearance rate correlated with the number of islets transplanted (Robertson et al., 2001). Another study showed reduced functional β-cell secretory reserve in IAT recipients, as compared with healthy individuals (Teuscher et al., 1998). Still another study showed that intrahepatic islet grafts failed to secrete glucagon in response to sustained hypoglycemia, but did in response to arginine, a peculiarity that may be site-dependent (Kendall et al., 1997). However, a study in dogs by another group indicated that alpha cell function was normal in the liver but not the omentum and spleen (Gustavson et al., 2005), so there are contradictory results Nonetheless, intraportal islet autografts at least release of insulin appropriately (Pyzdrowski et al., 1992).

In regard to IAT durability, there are case reports in which a long-functioning graft failed when the patient was given steroids for some reason, and often not an essential reason, with glucose toxicity killing the beta cells before it was realized that insulin to protect the stressed islets needed to be given (Ngo et al., 2011). Steroids should nearly never be administered to an IAT recipient. If there is a compelling reason to do so, insulin must be started or increased the moment steroids are begun in order to maintain euglycemia.

It should also be mentioned that exocrine deficiency can be a serious problem after TP, with or without an IAT (Stauffer et al., 2009), and unpredictable absorption can make diabetic management more difficult (Bellin et al., 2009). Exocrine deficiency has more of an impact on diabetic management after TP in those who do not than those that do have an IAT, especially those who are insulin-independent. Patients rank exocrine deficiency more of a problem than endocrine deficiency after TP-IAT (Braganza et al., 2011; Sutherland et al., 2011b).

13. Quality of life and pain relief

Health-related QOL is significantly worse in patients who have CP, as compared with a gender- and age-adjusted general population (Berney et al, 2000). The primary goal in performing TP-IAT is to improve QOL by alleviating pain and giving patients a chance to discontinue narcotics, while preventing or minimizing surgical diabetes. Studies evaluating health-related QOL outcomes after TP-IAT have been recently published. In reports from Cincinnati, QOL as measured by a standard assessment tool (SF-36) showed significant improvement a mean follow-up of .19 months (Rodriguez Rilo et al., 2003), and these findings were confirmed as more patients were included (Sutton et al., 2010).

Prospective studies of quality of life before and after TP-IAT have been conducted at the University Of Minnesota in both children (Bellin et al., 2011a) and adults (Bellin et al., 2011b). Both show significant improvement in QOL, as detailed above in the section on this institution.

As far as abdominal pain from CP that is refractory to high-dose narcotics, the Cincinatti group has published pain scores as assessed before after TP-IAT (Ahmad et al., 2005; Rodriguez Rilo et al., 2003). Narcotic independence was achieved in nearly two-thirds of patients after surgery, with a marked reduction in narcotic use by pre- and postoperative morphine-equivalent determinations (Ahmad et al., 2005).

These findings are similar to those in the University of Minnesota series with pain resolved or improved in nearly all and more than two-thirds able to eliminate narcotics while the remainder needed reduced doses (Bellin et al., 2011c;Carlson et al., 2007; Jie et al., 2005; Sutherland et al., 2009a; Sutherland et al., 2011b; Wahoff et al., 1995a) . Similar pain relief statistics are reported for CP patients undergoing TP without IAT (Behrman & Mulloy, 2006; Casadei et al., 2010b; Stauffer et al., 2009).

The patients who cannot withdraw completely from narcotics after TP usually have opioid-induced hyperalgesia (OIH) (Angst & Clark, 2006) from long term use prior to the surgery, a reason to not delay once it is apparent that a patient needs narcotics for pain in spite of other measures to treat the CP. Patients with OIH, are paradoxically become more sensitive to pain, by means of mechanisms originating in afferent neurons and in the spinal cord (Angst & Clark, 2006; Chuet al., 2006; Dogrul et al, 2005; Gardell et al, 2006; Liang et al, 2006; Mercadante , 2005). OIH may be highly prevalent in patients with long-standing CP and on narcotics for years before being referred for TP-IAT; accordingly, an endpoint such as narcotic independence may not be ideal for assessing postoperative success.

14. Cancer risk of chronic pancreatitis patients

The association between longstanding CP and cancer has been established (Ahmad et al., 2006; Braganza et al., 2011; Farrow & Evers , 2002; Lowenfels et al., 1993; Whitcomb & Pogue-Geile , 2002; Whitcomb, 2004). It is believed that pancreatic cancer develops in the setting of CP, independent of the underlying etiology, but appears to require 30 to 40 years of inflammation before manifesting in an appreciable percentage of patients (Whitcomb, 2004). This increased risk for pancreatic cancer is potentiated by cofactors such as tobacco and likely by genetic factors that are not yet entirely identified (Whitcomb & Pogue-Geile, 2002; Whitcomb DC, 2004).

A TP by itself for CP completely eliminates the risk of pancreatic cancer, but even with an IAT, the risk is lowered considerably, given the marked reduction in pancreatic tissue. The autologous islets infused into the portal system are never totally pure, but the use of tissue at risk for pancreatic cancer must be minimal. Sampling the whole gland for pathologic testing is impossible in the setting of an IAT. Patients who have hereditary and tropical pancreatitis are at higher risk for developing malignant cells than the rest of CP population (Farrow & Evers, 2002; Whitcomb DC, 2004) but again the amount of residual pancreatic tissue after TP-IAT is very small.

In the entire series of TP-IAT patients from UMN, no patients are known to have developed cancer in the liver or in any other site where the islets were auto-grafted, so the risk of cancer appears to be extremely low. In one case of IAT after a TP for pancreatic adenocarcinoma, cancer was not found in the liver at an autopsy two years later in which the patient died with metastatic disease elsewhere (Forster et al., 2004). Thus, the risk of pancreatic cancer developing in a liver after IAT when the TP is done for benign disease, including genetically linked CP (Sutton et al., 2010), is likely very low.

15. Future directions

A basic but important limitation to more widespread clinical application of IATs is the limited number of centers with the facilities and technology to isolate and prepare human islets. Few centers, including the authors', have used distance processing for both allogenic and autologous islets successfully (Langer et al., 2004; Rabkin et al., 1999; Rabkin et al., 1997). The feasibility of distance processing is enhanced by new preservation methods that extend cold ischemic times and increase islet yield and viability from suboptimal organs (Farrow & Evers, 2002; Fraker et al., 2002; Fujino et al., 1991; Langer et al, 2004; Lowenfels et al., 1993; Liang et al, 2006; Matsuda et al, 2003; Matsumoto, 2011; Mercadante,2005; Rabkin et al., 1997; Rabkin et al., 1999; Tsujimura et al., 2004; Tsujimura Tet al, 2004b; Whitcomb, 2004; Whitcomb & Pogue-Geile, 2002).

The long-term success of IATs in patients who have CP (Robertson et al., 2001) contrasts with the apparently less favorable long-term results for islet allotransplants in patients who have type 1 diabetes mellitus (Jahansouz et al., 2011; Ryan et al., 2005; Sabeck et al., 2009; Sutherland et al., 2008;), though in some center durable function does occur (Bellin et al., 2008b). The difference in outcomes may be because of the rejection rate of islet allografts, or if allografts are not rejected, to the diabetogenic effect of the necessary immunosuppression (Jahansouz et al., 2011).

Autologous islets are as fresh as possible. They are isolated from a pancreas that, although diseased, is not under the stress of brain death (which in animal models decreases islet yield and function by the activation of proinflammatory cytokines that occurs from central nervous system (CNS) injury (Contreras et al, 2003). A native pancreas removed for IAT also is not subjected to prolonged ischemia or to hours of cold preservation that occur with deceased donor pancreases processed for allogenic islets.

Single-donor islet allografts have resulted in insulin independence in diabetic recipients at UMN (Bellin et al., 2008b; Hering et al., 2005); yet in many cases, multiple donors are required (Jahansouz et al., 2011; Sutherland et al., 2004b). Increasing islet viability for transplants is important; for allografts, one possibility is to use a living donor (Matsumoto et al., 2005; Sutherland et al., 1980a; Sutherland et al., 1980b). This approach should be effective, given the good outcomes in IAT recipients with an islet mass well below that required for a successful outcome with deceased donor islet allografts (Sutherland, 2005; Sutherland et al., 2008).

A comparison of outcomes for IAT and ilset allogfafts provides an opportunity to distinguish between immunologic and nonimmunologic factors that affect declines in, or sustenance of, islet graft function over time. Whatever the variables, it is apparent that currently IATs are more successful than their allogenic counterparts (Sutherland et al., 2008)

16. Summary

TP-IAT has been used to treat painful CP for over 30 years. IAT is safe and prevents or minimizes surgical diabetes after TP for CP or even neoplastic disease in which a nondiseased portion of the pancreas can be used for islet isolation. Pancreatic resection (even partial) with an IAT always should be considered the primary surgical option for patients who have CP and intractable pain refractory to medical or endoscopic therapy. Pain relief, enabling narcotic discontinuation, is the primary objective; the prevention of diabetes is a secondary goal. The series reviewed here show that both goals are achieved to a reasonable degree in a very difficult disease, CP.

17. References

Ahmad, S., Lowy, A., Wray, C., D'Alessio, D., Choe, K., James, L. et al. (2005). Factors associated with insulin and narcotic independence after islet autotransplantation in patients with severe chronic pancreatitis. *J Am Coll Surg* Vol. 201, Issue 5, pp.680-687.

Ahmad, S., Wray, C., Rilo, H., & et.al. (2006). Chronic pancreatitis: recent advances and ongoing challenges. *Curr Probl Surg*, Vol. 43, pp. 127-238.

Anazawa, T., Balamurugan, A., Bellin, M., Zhang, H., Matsumoto, S., Yonekawa, Y. et al. (2009). Human islet isolation for autologous transplantation: comparison of yield and function using SERVA/Nordmark versus Roche enzymes. *Am J Transplant*, Vol. 9, Issue 10, pp. 2383-2391.

Anderson A, Korsgren O, & Jansson L. (1989). Intraportally transplanted pancreatic islets revascularized from hepatic arterial system. *Diabetes*, Vol. 38 Suppl 1, pp. 192-195.

Andren-Sandberg, A., Hoem, D., & Gislason, H. (2002). Pain management in chronic pancreatitis. *Eur J Gastroenterol Hepatol*, Vol. 14, 957-970.

Angst MS & Clark JD. (2006). Opioid-induced hyperalgesia: a qualitative systematic review. *Anesthesiology*. Vol. 104, Issue 3, pp. 570-587

Ao Z, Matayoshi K, Lakey JR, & et al. (1993). Survival and function of purified islets in the omental pouch site of outbred dogs. *Transplantation*, Vol. 56, Issue 3, pp. 524-529.

Argo, J., Contreras, J., Wesley, M., & Christein, J. (2008). Pancreatic resection with islet cell autotransplant for the treatment of severe chronic pancreatitis. *Am Surg*, Vol. 74, Issue 6, pp. 530-536.

Balamurugan, A. N., Bellin, M. D., Papas, K., Dunn, T. B., Vickers, S. M., Chinnakotla, S. et al. (2011a). Maximizing Islet Yield from Pancreata with Chronic Pancreatitis for Use in Islet Auto- Transplantation Requires a Modified Strategy from Islet Allograft Preparations. *Pancreas*, (in press).

Balamurugan, A. N., Soltani, S., Bellin, M., Sutliff, R., Loganathan, G., Papas, K. et al. (2011b) Naturally pure islets for autotransplantation after total pancreatectomy for chronic pancreatitis. *Xenotransplantation*, (in press).

Balamurugan, A. N., Wilhelm, J. J., Loganathan, G., Yuasa, T., Radosevich, D. M., Papas, K. et al. (2011c). Improved islet yield from diseased pancreases for autotransplantation using a new enzyme mixture. *American Journal of Transplantation*, (in press).

Behrman, S. & Mulloy, M. (2006). Total pancreatectomy for the treatment of chronic pancreatitis: indications, outcomes, and recommendations. *Am Surg*,Vol. 72, Issue 4, pp. 297-302.

Bellin, M. D., Carlson, A., Kobayashi, T., Gruessner, A., Hering, B., Moran, A. et al. (2007). Outcomes after pancreatectomy and autoislet transplantation in a pediatric population. *Xenotransplantation*, Vol. 14, Issue 5, p. 431.

Bellin, M. D., Carlson, A. M., Kobayashi, T., Gruessner, A. C., Hering, B. J., Moran, A. et al. (2008a). Outcome after pancreatectomy and islet autotransplantation in a pediatric population. *J.Pediatr.Gastroenterol.Nutr.,* Vol. 47, pp. 37-44.

Bellin, M. D., Kandaswamy, R., Parkey, J., Zhang, H. J., Liu, B., Ihm, S. H. et al. (2008b). Prolonged Insulin Independence After Islet Allotransplants in Recipients with Type 1 Diabetes. *Am.J.Transplant.,* Vol. *8,* pp. 2463-2470.

Bellin, M. D., Blondet, J. J., Beilman, G. J., Moran, A., Hering, B. J., & Sutherland, D. E. R. (2009). Islet function and glycemic control after total pancreatectomy and islet autotransplant. *Organ Biology,* Vol. 16, Issue 1, p. 122.

Bellin, M. D. & Sutherland, D. E. R. (2010). Pediatric Islet Autotransplantation: Indication, Technique, and Outcome. *Curr Diab Rep,* Vol. *10,* Issue 5, pp. 326-331.

Bellin, M. D., Blondet, J. J., Beilman, G. J., Dunn, T. B., Balamurugan, A. N., Thomas, W. et al. (2010a). Predicting islet yield in pediatric patients undergoing pancreatectomy and autoislet transplantation for chronic pancreatitis. *Pediatr.Diabetes,* Vol. 11, pp. 227-234.

Bellin, M. D., Freeman, M. L., Schwarzenberg, S. J., Radosevich, D. M., Dunn, T. B., Beilman, G. J. et al. (2010b). Quality of Life After Total Pancreatectomy and Islet Autotransplant for Chronic Pancreatitis in Children. *Pancreas,* Vol. 39, Issue 8, pp. 1310-1311.

Bellin, M., Moran, A., Hering, B. J., Chinnakotla, S., Balamurugan, A. N., Dunn, T. B. et al. (2011a). Islet autotransplant outcomes in thirty-six children undergoing pancreatectomy and islet autotransplant. *The Review of Diabetic Studies: Special IPITA Congress 2011 Issue on Pancreas and Islet Transplantation,* Vol. 8, Issue 1, p. 101.

Bellin, M. D., Freeman, M., Schwarzenberg, S., Dunn, T. B., Beilman, G. J., Vickers, S. M. et al. (2011b). Quality of Life Improves for Pediatric Patients After Total Pancreatectomy and Islet Autotransplant for Chronic Pancreatitis. *Clin Gastroenterol Hepatol,* (in press).

Bellin, M. D., Radosevich, D., Beilman, G., Dunn, T. B., Chinnakotla, S., Bland, B. et al. (2011c). Quality of life after pancreatectomy and islet autotransplant. *Pancreas,* (in press).

Berney T, Rudisuhli T, Oberholzer J, & et al. (2000). Long-term metabolic results after pancreatic resection for severe chronic pancreatitis. *Arch Surg,* Vol. 135, Issue 9, pp. 1106-1111.

Berney T, Mathe Z, Bucher P, & et al. (2004). Islet autotransplantation for the prevention of surgical diabetes after extended pancreatectomy for the resection of benign tumors of the pancreas. *Transplant Proc,* Vol. 36, Issue 4, pp. 1123-1124.

Billings, B., Christein, J., Harmsen, W., Harrington, J., Chari, S., Que, F. et al. (2011). Quality-of-life after total pancreatectomy: is it really that bad on long-term follow-up? *J Gastrointest Surg,* Vol. 9, Issue 8, pp. 1059-1066.

Blondet, J., Carlson, A., Kobayashi, T., Jie, T., Bellin, M., Hering, B. et al. (2007). The role of total pancreatectomy and islet autotransplantation for chronic pancreatitis. *Surg Clin N Am,* Vol. 87, Issue 6, 1477-1501.

Braganza, J., Lee, S., McCloy, R., & McMahon, M. (2011). Chronic pancreatitis. *Lancet,* Vol. 377, Issue 9772, pp. 1184-1197.

Buscher HC, Wilder-Smith OH, & van Goor H. (2006). Chronic pancreatitis patients show hyperalgesia of central origin: a pilot study. *Eur J Pain,* Vol. 10, Issue 4, pp. 363-370.

Cahen, D. L., Gouma, D. J., Nio, Y., & et al. (2007). Endoscopic versus surgical dainage of the pancreatic duct in chronic pancreatitis. *N. Engl .J.Med,* Vol. 356, Issue 7, pp. 676-684.

Cameron JL, Mehigan DG, Broe PJ, & Zuidema GD. (1981). Distal pancreatectomy and islet autotransplantation for chronic pancreatitis. *Ann Surg,* Vol. 193, Issue 3, pp. 312-317.

Carlson, A., Kobayashi, T., & Sutherland, D. E. R. (2007). Islet autotransplantation to prevent or minimize diabetes after pancreatectomy. *Curr Opinion in Organ Transplantation,* Vol. *12,* pp. 82-88.

Casadei, R., Marchegiani, G., Laterza, M., Ricci, C., Marrano, N., Margiotta, A. et al. (2009). Total pancreatectomy: doing it with a mini-invasive approach. *JOP,* Vol. 10, Issue 3, pp. 328-331.

Casadei, R., Monari, F., Buscemi, S., Laterza, M., Ricci, C., Rega, D. et al. (2010a). Total pancreatectomy: indications, operative technique, and results: a single centre experience and review of literature. *Updates Surg,* Vol. 62, Issue 1, pp. 41-46.

Casadei, R., Ricci, C., Monari, F., Laterza, M., Rega, D., D'Ambra, M. et al. (2010b). Clinical outcome of patients who underwent total pancreatectomy. *Pancreas,* Vol. 39, Issue 4, pp. 546-547.

Casey J.J., Lakey, J.R., Ryan, E.A., & et al. (2002). Portal venous pressure changes after sequential clinical islet transplantation. *Transplantation,* Vol. 74, Issue 7, pp. 913-915.

Chong AK, Hawes RH, Hoffman BJ, & et al. (2007). Diagnostic performance of EUS for chronic pancreatitis: a comparison with histopathology. *Gastrointest.Endos,* Vol. 65, pp. 808-814.

CITR Coordinating Center and Investigators (2009). *2009 Collaborative Islet Transplant Registry Annual Report.* http://www.citregistry.org/reports/reports.htm.

Clark A, Bown, E, King T, & et al. (1982). Islet changes induced by hyperglycemia in rats. Effect of insulin or chlorpropamide therapy. *Diabetes,* Vol. 31, Issue 4 Pt 1, pp. 319-325.

Clayton, H., Davies, J., Pollard, C., & et.al. (2003). Pancreatectomy with islet autotransplantation for the treatment of severe chronic pancreatitis: the first 40 patients at the Leicester General Hospital. *Transplantation,* Vol. 76, pp. 92-98.

Contreras JL, Eckstein C, Smyth CA, & et al. (2003). Brain death significantly reduces isolated pancreatic islet yields and functionality in vitro and in vivo after transplantation in rats. *Diabetes* Vol. 52, Issue 12, pp. 2935-2942.

Corlett MP & Scharp DW. (1998). The effect of pancreatic warm ischemia on islet isolation in rats and dogs. *J Surg Res,* Vol. 45, Issue 6, pp. 531-536.

Desai, C. S., Stephenson, D., Khalid, K. M., Jie, T., Gruessner, A. C., Rilo, H. L. et al. (2011). Novel technique of total pancreatectomy before autologous islet transplants in chronic pancreatitis patients. *J Am Coll Surg,* (in press).

Di Sebastiano, P., Fink, T., Weihe, E., & et al. (1997). Immune cell infiltration and growth-associated protein 43 expression correlate with pain in chronic pancreatitis. *Gastroenterology,* Vol. 112, Issue 5, pp. 1648-1655.

Di Sebastiano, P., Di Mola, F., Buchler, M., & Friess, H. (2004). Pathogenesis of pain in chronic pancreatitis. *Dig Dis,* Vol. 22, Issue 3, pp. 267-272.

Dite, P., Ruzicka, M., Zboril, V., & Novotny, I. (2003). A prospective, randomized trial comparing endoscopic and surgical therapy for chronic pancreatitis. *Endoscopy,* Vol. *35,* pp. 765-776.

Dixon, J., DeLegge, M., Morgan, K., & Adams, D. (2008). Impact of total pancreatectomy with islet cell transplant on chronic pancreatitis management at a disease-based center. *Am Surg,* Vol. 74, Issue 8, pp. 735-738.

Dohan FC & Lukens, FW. (1947). Lesions of the pancreatic islets produced in cats by the administration of glucose. *Science,* Vol. 105, Issue 183, p. 183.

Dong, M., Parksaik, A., Erwin, P., Farnell, M., Murad, M., & Kudva, Y. (2011) Systematic Review and Meta-analysis: Islet Autotransplantation after Pancreatectomy for Minimizing Diabetes. *Clin Endocrino Oxfl,* (in press).

Ekberg K, Brismar T, Johansson BL, & et al. (2003). Amelioration of sensory nerve dysfunction by C-Peptide in patients with type 1 diabetes. *Diabetes* Vol. 52, Issue 2, pp. 536-541

Etemad, B. & Whitcomb, D. C. (2001). Chronic pancreatitis: diagnosis, classification, and new genetic developments. *Gastroenterology,* Vol. *120,* pp. 682-707.

Farkas, G. & Pap, A. (1997). Management of diabetes induced by nearly total (95%) pancreatectomy with autologous transplantation of Langerhans cells. *Orv Hetil,* Vol. 29, pp. 1863-1867.

Farney, A., Najarian, J., & Nakhleh, R. (1991). Autotransplantation of dispersed pancreatic islet tissue combined with total or near-total pancreatectomy for treatment of chronic pancreatitis. *Surgery,* Vol. 110, pp. 427-439.

Farney, A. C., Hering, B. J., Nelson, L. A., Tanioka, Y., Gilmore, T., Leone, J. P. et al. (1998). No late failures of intraportal human islet autografts beyond 2 years. *Transplant Proc,* Vol. 30, p. 420.

Farney, A. C. & Sutherland, D. E. (2008). A quick look back at the history of pancreatic surgery. *Ann.Surg., Vol. 248,* pp. 498-499.

Fasanella, K. E., Davis, B., Lyons, J., & et al. (2007). Pain in chronic pancreatitis and pancreatic cancer. *Gastroenterol Clin N Am,* Vol. *36,* pp. 335-364.

Fontana I, Arcuri V, Tommasi GV, & et al. (1994). Long-term follow-up of human islet autotransplantation. *Transplant Proc,* Vol. 26, Issue 2, p. 581.

Forster S, Liu X, Adam U, & et al. (2004). Islet autotransplantation combined with pancreatectomy for treatment of pancreatic adenocarcinoma: a case report. *Transplant Proc,* Vol. 36, Issue 4, pp. 1125- 1126.

Fujino Y, Matsumoto I, Ajiki T, & Kuroda Y. (2009). Clinical reappraisal of total pancreatectomy for pancreatic disease. *Pancreas,* Vol. 56, Issue 94-95, pp. 1525- 1528.

Fukushima W, Shimizu K, Izumi R, & et al. (1994). Heterotopic segmental pancreatic autotransplantation in patients undergoing total pancreatectomy. *Transplant Proc,* Vol. 26, Issue 4, pp. 2285-2287.

Gachago, C. & Draganov, P. (2008). Pain management in chronic pancreatitis. *World J Gastroenterol,* Vol. 14, Issue 20, pp. 3137-3148.

Garcea, G., Weaver, J., Phillips, J., Pollard, C., Ilouz, S., Webb, M. et al. (2009). Total pancreatectomy with and without islet cell transplantation for chronic pancreatitis: a series of 85 consectuive patients. *Pancreas,* Vol. 38, Issue 1, p. 1-7.

Giulianotti, P., Kuechle, H., Salehi, P., Gorodner, V., Galvani, C., Benedetti, E. et al. (2009). Robotic-assisted laparoscopic distal pancreatectomy of a redo case combined with autologous islet transplantation for chronic pancreatitis. *Pancreas,* Vol. 38, Issue 1, pp. 105-107.

Giulianotti, P., Addeo, P., Buchs, N., Bianco, F., & Ayloo, S. (2011). Early experience with robotic total pancreatectomy. *Pancreas,* Vol. 40, Issue 2, pp. 311-313.

Gores, P. F., Najarian, J. S., & Sutherland, D. E. R. (1992). Islet Autotransplantation. In: *Pancreatic Islet Cell Transplantation,* C. Ricordi (Ed.), pp. 291-312 R.G. Landers Company, Austin.

Gores, PF & Sutherland, DE. (1993). Pancreatic islet transplantation: is purification necessary? *Am J Surg,* Vol. 166, Issue 5, pp. 538-542.

Gray DW, Sutton R, McShane P, & et al. (1988). Exocrine contamination impairs implantation of pancreatic islets transplanted beneath the kidney capsule. *J Surg Res,* Vol. 45, pp. 432-442.

Gray DW, Cranston D, McShane P, & et al. (1989). The effect of hyperglycaemia on pancreatic islets transplanted into rats beneath the kidney capsule. *Diabetologia,* Vol. 32, Issue 9, pp. 663-667.

Gray DW. (1990). Islet isolation and transplantation techniques in the primate. *Surg Gynecol Obstet,* Vol. 170, Issue 3, pp. 225-232.

Greenway SE, Greenway FL, 3., & Klein S. (2002). Effects of obesity surgery on non-insulin-dependent diabetes mellitus. *Arch Surg,* Vol. 137, Issue 10, pp. 1109-1117.

Gruessner, R. W., Sutherland, D. E., Dunn, D. L., Najarian, J. S., Jie, T., Hering, B. J. et al. (2004). Transplant options for patients undergoing total pancreatectomy for chronic pancreatitis. *J Am Coll Surg,* Vol. *198,* pp. 559-567; discussion 568-9.

Gruessner, R., Sutherland, D., Drangstveit, M., Kandaswamy, R., & Gruessner, A. (2008). Pancreas allotransplants in patients with a previous total pancreatectomy for chronic pancreatitis. *J Am Coll Surg,* Vol. 206, Issue 3, pp. 458-465.

Grunkemeier, D. M. S., Cassara, J. E., Dalton, C. B., & Drossman, D. A. (2007). The Narcotic Bowel Syndrome: Clinical Features, Pathophysiology, and Management. *Clin Gastroenterol Hepatol,* Vol. 5, pp. 1126-1139.

Gupta, K., Carlson, A., & Kobayashi, T. (2007). EUS in early chronic pancreatitis: Comparison with histopathology in patients undergoing total pancreatectomy with autologous islet cell transplantation. In *Digestive Disease Week,* Washington, DC.

Gustavson, S., Rajotte, R., Hunkeler, D., Lakey, J., Edgerton, D., Neal, D. et al. (2005). Islet auto-t ransplantation into an omental or splenic site results in a normal beta cell but abnormal alpha cell response to mild non-insulin-induced hypoglycemia. *Am J Transplant,* Vol. 5, Issue 10, pp. 2368- 2377.

Heidt, D., Burant, C., & Simeone, D. (2007). Total pancreatectomy: indications, operative technique, and postoperative sequelae. J Gastrointest Surg 11[2], 209-216.

Hering BJ, Wijkstrom M, & Eckman PM (2004). Islet transplantation. In: *Transplantation of the Pancreas,* Gruessner RW & Sutherland DER (Eds.), pp. 583-626, Springer-Verlag, New York.

Hering, B. J., Kandaswamy, R., Ansite, J., Eckman, P., Nakano, M., Sawada, T. et al. (2005). Single-donor, marginal-dose islet transplantation in patients with type 1 diabetes. *JAMA,* Vol. *293,* pp. 830-835.

Hermann, M., Margeiter, R., & Hengster, P. (2010). Human Islet Autotransplantation: The Trail Thus Far and the Highway Ahead. *Adv Exp Med Biol* , Vol. 654, pp. 711-724.

Hinshaw, D. B., Jolley, W. B., Hinshaw, D., Kaiser, J. E., & Hinshaw, K. (2011). Islet Autotransplantation After Pancreatectomy for Chronic Pancreatitis With a New Method of Islet Preparation. *Am J Surg,* Vol. 42, pp. 118-122.

Hogle HH & Recemtsma K. (1978). Pancreatic autotransplantation following resection. *Surgery,* Vol. 83, Issue 3, pp. 359-360.

Jahansouz, C., Jahansouz, C., Kumer, S., & Brayman, K. (2011). Evolution of ß-Cell Replacement Therapy in Diabetes Mellitus: Islet Cell Transplantation. *Journal of Transplantation,* (in press).

Janot, M., Belyaev, O., Kersting, S., Chromik, A., Seelig, M., Sulberg, D. et al. (2010). Indications and early outcomes for total pancreatectomy at a high-volume pancreas center. *HPB Surg,* Article ID 686702.

Jethwa, P., Sodergren, M., Lala, A., Webber, J., Buckels, J., Bramhall, S. et al. (2006). Diabetic control after total pancreatectomy. *Dig Liver Dis,* Vol. 38, Issue 6, pp. 415-419.

Jie, T., Hering, B. J., Ansite, J. D., Gilmore, T. R., Fraga, D. W., & Beilman, G. J. (2005). Pancreatectomy and auto-islet transplant in patients with chronic pancreatitis. *J. Am .Coll. Surg.,* Vol. *201,* p. S14.

Jindal, R., Finebergm, S., & et al. (1998). Clinical experience with autologous and allogeneic pancreatic islet transplantation. *Transplantation,* Vol. 66, Issue 12, pp. 1836-1841.

Johansson BL, Borg K, Fernqvist-Forbes E, & et al. (2000). Beneficial effects of C-peptide on incipient nephropathy and neuropathy in patients with Type 1 diabetes mellitus. *Diabet Med* , Vol. 17, Issue 3, pp. 181-189.

Jung, H. S., Choi, S. H., Kim, S. J., Choi, D. W., Heo, J., Lee, K. T. et al. (2009). Delayed improvement of insulin secretion after autologous islet transplantation in partially pancreatectomized pati. *Metabolism,* Vol. 58, Issue 11, pp. 1629-1635.

Kahl, S., Glasbrenner, B., Zimmerman, S., & et al. (2002). Endoscopic ultrasound in pancreatic diseases. *Dig Dis,* Vol. *20,* pp. 120-126.

Kamiya H, Zhang W, & Sima AA. (2004). C-peptide prevents nociceptive sensory neuropathy in type 1 diabetes. *Ann Neurol,* Vol. 56, Issue 6, pp 827-835.

Keith RG, Keshavjee SH, & Kerenyi NR. (1985). Neuropathology of chronic pancreatitis in humans. *Can J Surg,* Vol. 28, Issue 3, pp. 207-211.

Kendall DM, Teuscher AU, & Robertson RP. (1997). Defective glucagon secretion during sustained hypoglycemia following successful islet allo- and autotransplantation in humans. *Diabetes,* Vol. 46, pp. 23-27.

Kobayashi, T., Manivel, J., Bellin, M., Carlson, A., Moran, A., Freeman, M. L. et al. (2010). Correlation of pancreatic histopathologic findings and islet yield in children with chronic pancreatitis undergoing total pancreatectomy and islet autotransplantation. *Pancreas,* Vol. 39, Issue 1, pp. 57-63.

Kobayashi, T., Manivel, J. C., Carlson, A. M., Bellin, M. D., Moran, A., Freeman, M. L. et al. (2011). Correlation of Histopathology, Islet Yield, and Islet Graft Function After Islet Autotransplantation in Chronic Pancreatitis. *Pancreas,* Vol. 40, Issue 2, pp. 193-199.

Korsgren O, Jansson L, & Andersson A. (1989). Effects of hyperglycemia on function of isolated mouse pancreatic islets transplanted under kidney capsule. *Diabetes,* Vol. 38, Issue 4, pp. 510-515.

Korsgren O, Christofferson R, & Jansson L. (1999). Angiogenesis and angioarchitecture of transplanted fetal porcine islet-like cell clusters. *Transplantation,* Vol. 68, Issue 11, pp. 1761-1766.

Koukoutsis, I., Tamijmarane, A., Bellagamba, R., Bramhall, S., Buckels, J., & Mirza, D. (2007). The impact of splenectomy on outcomes after distal and total pancreatectomy. *World J Surg Oncol*, Vol. 2, Issue 5, p. 61.

Langer RM, Mathe Z, Doros A, & et al. (2004). Successful islet after kidney transplantations in a distance over 1000 kilometers: Preliminary results of the Budapest-Geneva collaboration. *Transplant Proc.*, Vol. 36, Issue 10, pp. 3113-3115.

Layer, P., Yamamoto, H., Kalthoff, L., Clain, J. E., Bakken, L. J., & DiMagno, E. P. (1994). The different courses of early- and late-onset idiopathic and alcoholic chronic pancreatitis. *Gastroenterology*, Vol. 107, pp. 1481-1487.

le Roux CW, Aylwin SJ, Batterham RL, & et al. (2006). Gut hormone profiles following bariatric surgery favor an anorectic state, facilitate weight loss, and improve metabolic parameters. *Ann Surg*, Vol. 242, pp. 108-114.

Lee BW, Jee JH, Heo JS, & et al. (2005). The favorable outcome of human islet transplantation in Korea: experiences of 10 autologous transplantations. *Transplantation*, Vol. 79, Issue 11, pp. 1568-1574.

Leone, J. P., Kendall, D. M., Reinsmoen, N. L., Hering, B. J., & Sutherland, D. E. R. (1998). Immediate insulin-independence after retransplantation of islets prepared from an allograft pancreatectomy in a Type I diabetic patient. *Transplant. Proc.*, Vol. 30, Issue 2, p. 319.

Maisonneuve, P., Lowenfels, A. B., Mullhaupt, B., & et al. (2005). Cigarette smoking accelerates progression of alcoholic chronic pancreatitis. *Gut*, Vol. *54*, pp. 510-514.

Makhlouf L, Duvivier-Kali VF, Bonner-Weir S, & et al. (2003). Importance of hyperglycemia on the primary function of allogenic islet transplants. *Transplantation*, Vol. 76, pp. 657-664.

Manciu N, Beebe DS, Tran P, & et al. (1999). Total pancreatectomy with islet cell autotransplantation: anesthetic implications. *J Clin Anesth*, Vol. 11, Issue 7, pp. 576-582.

Manes G, Buchler M, Pieramico O, & et al. (1994). Is increased pancreatic pressure related to pain in chronic pancreatitis? *Int J Pancreatol*, Vol. 15, Issue 2, pp. 113-117.

Marquez, S., Marquez, T. T., Ikramuddin, S., Kandaswamy, R., Antanavicius, G., Freeman, M. L. et al. (2010). Laparoscopic and da Vinci robot-assisted total pancreatectomy, duodenectomy, and islet auto transplantation: Case report of a definitive minimally invasive treatment for chronic pancreatitis. *Pancreas*, Vol. *39*, pp. 1109-1111.

Matarazzo M, Giardina MG, Guardasole V, & et al. (2002). Islet transplantation under the kidney capsule corrects the defects in glycogen metabolism in both liver and muscle of streptozocin-diabetic rats. *Cell Transplant*, Vol. 11, Issue 2, pp. 103-112.

Matsumoto, S., Okitsu, T., Iwanaga, Y., Noguchi, H., Nagata, H., Yonekawa, Y. et al. (2005). Insulin- independence of unstable diabetic patient after single living-donor islet transplantation. *Transplant Proc*, Vol. 3., Issue 8, pp. 3427-3429.

Matsumoto, S. (2011). Autologous Islet Cell Transplantation to Prevent Surgical Diabetes. *J Diabetes*, (in press).

Mehigan DG, Bell WR, Zuidema GD, & et al. (1980). Disseminated intravascular coagulation and portal hypertension following pancreatic islet autotransplantation. *Ann Surg*, Vol. 191, Issue 3, pp. 287- 293.

Memsic L, Busuttil RW, & Traverso LW. (1984). Bleeding esophageal varices and portal vein thrombosis after pancreatic mixed-cell autotransplantation. *Surgery,* Vol. 95, Issue 2, pp. 238-242.

Morgan, K., Nishimura, M., Uflacker, R., & Adams, D. (2011). Percutaneous transhepatic islet cell autotransplantation after pancreatectomy for chronic pancreatitis: a novel approach. *HPB (Oxford),* Vol. 13, Issue 7, pp. 1477-2574.

Morrow, C. E., Cohen, J. I., Sutherland, D. E. R., & Najarian, J. S. (1984). Chronic pancreatitis: Long-term surgical results of pancreatic duct drainage, pancreatic resection, and near-total pancreatectomy and islet autotransplantation. *Surgery., 96,* 608-616.

Muller, M., Friess, H., Kleef, J., Dahmen, R., Wagner, M., Hinz, U. et al. (2007). Is there still a role for total pancreatectomy? *Ann Surg,* Vol. 246, Issue 6, pp. 966-974.

Mullhaupt, B. & Ammann, R. W. (2010). Total pancreatectomy for intractable pain in chronic pancreatitis? *Pancreas,* Vol. 39, Issue 1, pp. 111-112.

Murphy, M., Knaus, W., Ng, S., Hill, J., McPhee, J., Shah, S. et al. (2009). Total pancreatectomy: a national study. *HPB (Oxford),* Vol. 11, Issue, 6, pp. 476-482.

Najarian, J. S., Sutherland, D. E. R., Matas, A. J., Steffes, M. W., Simmons, R. L., & Goetz, F. C. (1977). Human islet transplantation: A preliminary experience. *Transplant.Proc.,* Vol. *9,* pp.233-236.

Najarian, J. S., Sutherland, D. E. R., Matas, A. J., & Goetz, F. C. (1979). Human islet autotransplantation following pancreatectomy. *Transplant. Proc.,* Vol. 11, Issue 1, pp. 336-340.

Najarian, J. S., Sutherland, D. E. R., Baumgartner, D., Burke, B., Rynasiewicz, J. J., Matas, A. J. et al. (1980). Total or near total pancreatectomy and islet autotransplantation for treatment of chronic pancreatitis. *Ann.Surg., 192,* 526-542.

Nath, D., Kellogg, T., & Sutherland, D. (2004). Total pancreatectomy with intraportal auto-islet transplantation using a temporarily exteriorized omental vein. *J Am Coll Surg,* Vol. 199, Issue 6, pp. 994-995.

Ngo, A., Sutherland, D., Beilman, G., & Bellin, M. (2011). Deterioration of glycemic control after corticosteroid administration in islet autotransplant recipients: a cautionary tale. *Acta Diabetol.,* (in press).

Noh KW & Wallace, M. (2006). EUS in the Diagnosis of Chronic Pancreatitis. *Visible Human Journal of Endoscopy,* Vol. 5, Issue 1, pp. 6-8.

Oberholzer, J., Triponez, F., Mage, R., & et al. (2000). Human islet transplantation: lessons from 13 autologous and 13 allogeneic transplantations. *Transplantation,* Vol. 69, Issue 6, pp. 1115-1123.

Oberholzer J, Mathe Z, Bucher P, & et al. (2003). Islet autotransplantation after left pancreatectomy for non- enucleable insulinoma. *Am J Transplant ,* Vol. 3, Issue 10, pp. 1302-1307.

Onaca, N., Naziruddin, B., Matsumoto, S., Noguchi, H., Klintmalm, G., & Levy, M. (2007). Pancreatic islet cell transplantation: update and new developments. *Nutr Clin Pract,* Vol. 22, Issue 5, pp. 485-493.

Ong, S., Pollard, C., Rees, Y., Garcea, G., Webb, M., Illouz, S. et al. (2008). Ultrasound changes within the liver after total pancreatectomy and intrahepatic islet cell autotransplantation. *Transplantation,* Vol. 85, Issue 12, pp. 1773-1777.

Papas, K. K., Bellin, M., Sutherland, D. E., Mueller, K., Avgoustiniatos, E. S., Balamurugan, A. N. et al. (2010). Viable Islet Dose Based on Oxygen Consumption Rate Predicts Clinical Islet Autotransplant Outcome: 2010. *Transplantation,* Vol 90, p. 137.

Parsaik, A., Murad, M., Sathananthan, A., Moorthy, V., Erwin, P., Chari, S. et al. (2010). Metabolic and target organ outcomes after total pancreatectomy: Mayo Clinic experience and meta-analysis of the literature. *Clin Endocrinol,* Vol. 73, Issue 6, pp. 723-731.

Pezzilli, R. (2006). Diabetic control after total pancreatectomy. *Dig Liver Dis,* Vol. 38, Issue 6, pp. 415-419.

Pollard, C., Gravante, G., Webb, M., Chung, W., Illouz, S., Ong, S. et al. (2011). Use of the Recanalised Umbilical Vein for Islet Autotransplantation following Total Pancreatectomy. *Pancreatology,* Vol. 11, Issue 2, pp. 233-239.

Pyzdrowski, K. L., Kendall, D. M., Halter, J. B., Nakhleh, R. E., Sutherland, D. E. R., & Robertson, R. P. (1992). Preserved insulin secretion and insulin independence in recipients of islet autografts. *New Engl. J. Med.,* Vol. 327, Issue 4, pp. 220-226.

Rabkin, J. M., Leone, J. P., Sutherland, D. E. R., Ahman, A., Reed, M., Papalois, B. et al. (1997). Transcontinental shipping of pancreatic islets for autotransplantation after total pancreatectomy. *Pancreas,* Vol. *15,* pp. 416-419.

Rabkin, J. M., Olyaei, A. J., Orloff, S. L., Geisler, S. M., Wahoff, D. C., Hering, B. J. et al. (1999). Distant processing of pancreas islets for autotransplantation following total pancreatectomy. *Am.J.Surg.,* Vol. *177,* pp. 423-427.

Rafael, E., Tibell, A., Ryden, M., Lundgren, T., Savendahl, L., Borgstrom, B. et al. (2008). Intramuscular autotransplantation of pancreatic islets in a 7-year-old child: a 2-year follow-up. *Am. J. Transplant,* Vol. 8, pp. 458-462.

Rajab, A., Buss, J., Diakoff, E., Hadley, G., Osei, K., & Ferguson, R. (2008). Comparison of the portal vein and kidney subcapsule as sites for primate islet autotransplantation. *Cell Transplant,* Vol. 17, Issue 9, pp. 1015-1023.

Rastellini, C., Brown, M., & Circalese, L. (2006). Heparin-induced thrombocytopenia following pancreatectomy and islet auto-transplantation. *Clin Transplant,* Vol. 20, Issue 2, pp. 156-158.

Ris, F., Niclauss, N., Morel, P., Demuylder, S., Muller, Y., Meier, R. et al. (2011). Islet Autotransplantation After Extended Pancreatectomy for Focal Benign Disease of the Pancreas. *Transplantation,* Vol. 91, Issue 8, pp. 895-901.

Robertson RP. (2001). Pancreatic islet cell transplantation: likely impact on current therapeutics for type 1 diabetes mellitus. *Drugs,* Vol. 61, Issue 14, pp. 2017-2020.

Robertson, R. P., Lanz, K. J., Sutherland, D. E., & Kendall, D. M. (2001). Prevention of diabetes for up to 13 years by autoislet transplantation after pancreatectomy for chronic pancreatitis. *Diabetes,* Vol. 50, pp. 47-50.

Robertson, P. R. (2010a). Islet Transplantation a Decade Later and Strategies for Filling a Half-Full Glass. *Diabetes,* Vol. 59, pp. 185-191.

Robertson, P. R. (2010b). Update on Transplanting Beta Cells for Reversing Type 1 Diabetes. *Endocrinol Metab Clin N,* Vol. 39, pp. 665-667.

Rodriguez Rilo, H., Ahmad, S., D'Alessio, D., & et.al. (2003). Total pancreatectomy and autologous islet cell transplantation as a means to treat severe chronic pancreatitis. *J Gastrointest Surg,* Vol. 7, pp. 978- 989.

Rossi RL, Soeldner JS, Braasch JW, & et al. (1986). Segmental pancreatic autotransplantation with pancreatic ductal occlusion after near total or total pancreatic resection for chronic pancreatitis. *Ann Surg*, Vol. 203, pp. 626-636.

Ryan EA, Paty BW, Senior PA, & et al. (2005). Five-year follow-up after clinical islet transplantation. *Diabetes*, Vol. 54, Issue 7, pp. 2060-2069.

Sabeck, O., Hamilton, D., & Gaber, A. (2009). Prospects for future advancements in islet cell transplantation. *Minerva Chir.* Vol. 64, Issue 1, pp. 59-73.

Sahai, A. V., Zimmerman, M., Aabakken, L., Tarnasky, P. R., Cunningham, J. T., van, V. A. et al. (1998). Prospective assessment of the ability of endoscopic ultrasound to diagnose, exclude, or establish the severity of chronic pancreatitis found by endoscopic retrograde cholangiopancreatography. *Gastrointest.Endosc.*, Vol. 48, pp. 18-25.

Sakata, N., Egawa, S., Motoi, F., Mikami, Y., Ishida, M., Aoki, T. et al. (2008). Institutional indications for islet transplantation after total pancreatectomy. *J Hepatobiliary Pancreat Surg*, Vol. 15, Issue 5, pp. 488-492.

Sarbu, V., Dima, S., Aschie, M., & et al. (2005). Preliminary data on post-pancreatectomy diabetes mellitus treated by islet-cell autotransplantation. *Chirurg.(Bucur)*, Vol. 100, Issue 587, p. 593.

Schneider, A. & Whitcomb, D. C. (2002). Hereditary pancreatitis: a model for inflammatory diseases of the pancreas. *Best Pract Res Clin Gastroenterol*, Vol. *16*, pp. 347-363.

Schmulewitz, N. Total Pancreatectomy With Autologous Islet Cell Transplantation in Children: Making a Difference (2011). *Clin Gastroenterol.Hepatol.*, (in press).

Simons, J., Shah, S., Ng, S., Whalen, G., & Tseng, J. (2009). National complication rates after pancreatectomy: beyond mere mortality. *J Gastrointest Surg*, Vol. 13, Issue 10, pp. 1798-1805.

Soltani, S., Loganathan, G., Bellin, M., Papas, K., Dunn, T., Vickers, S. et al. (2011a). Reducing the transplantable tissue volume for human islet auto-transplantation: A high density purification process different from islet allograft purification. *The Review of Diabetic Studies: Special IPITA Congress 2011 Issue on Pancreas and Islet Transplantation*, Vol. 8, Issue 1, pp. 149-150.

Soltani, S., Loganathan, G., Bellin, M. D., Tiwari, M., Papas, K., Vickers, S. et al. (2011b) Islet isolation outcome from minimal change chronic pancreatitis is comparable with clinical grade allograft pancreases. *American Journal of Transplantation*, (in press).

Soltani, S. M., O'Brien, T. D., Loganathan, G., Bellin, M. D., Anazawa, T., Tiwari, M. et al. (2011c). Severely fibrotic pancreases from young patients with chronic pancreatitis: evidence for a ductal origin of islet neogenesis. *Acta Diabetol.*, (in press).

Stauffer, J., Nguyen, J., Heckman, M., Grewal, M., Dougherty, M., Gill, K. et al. (2009). Patient outcomes after total pancreatectomy: a single centre contemporary experience. *HPB (Oxford)*, Vol. 11, Issue 6, pp. 483-492.

Sutherland, D. E. R., Matas, A. J., & Najarian, J. S. (1978). Pancreatic islet cell transplantation. *Surg.Clin.No.Amer.*, Vol. *58*, pp. 365-382.

Sutherland, D. E. R., Matas, A. J., Goetz, F. C., & Najarian, J. S. (1980a). Transplantation of dispersed pancreatic islet tissue in humans: autografts and allografts. *Diabetes*, Vol. 29 (Suppl. 1*)*, pp. 31-44.

Sutherland, D. E., Goetz, F. C., & Najarian, J. S. (1980b). Living-related donor segmental pancreatectomy for transplantation. *Transplant Proc*, Vol. *12*, pp. 19-25.

Sutherland, D. E. R., Gruessner, R. G., Jie, T., Nath, D., Sielaff, T., Dunn, D. L. et al. (2004a). Pancreatic islet auto-transplantation for chronic pancreatitis. *Clinical Transplantation*, Vol. 18, Issue Supplement 13, pp. 17-18.

Sutherland, D. E. R., Gruessner, A., & Hering, J. (2004b). Beta-cell replacement therapy (pancreas and islet transplantation): an integrated approach. *Endocr. Metab. Clin. N. Amer., Vol.* 33, pp. 135-148.

Sutherland, D. E. R. (2005). Beta-cell replacement by transplantation in diabetes mellitus: which patients at what risk, which way (when pancreas, when islets), and how to allocate deceased donor pancreases. *Curr Opinion in Organ Transplantation,* Vol. 10, pp. 147-149.

Sutherland, D., Gruessner, A., Carlson, A., Blondet, J., Balamurugan, A., Reigstad, K. et al. (2008). Islet autotransplant outcomes after total pancreatectomy: a contrast to islet allograft outcomes. *Transplantation*, Vol. 86, Issue 12, pp. 1799-1802.

Sutherland, D., Radosevich, D., Bland, B., Beilman, G., Dunn, T., Vickers, S. et al. (2009a). Total pancreatectomy (TP) and islet autotransplants (IAT) for chronic pancreatitis (CP): early outcomes in recent cases. *Pancreas,* Vol. 38, Issue 8, p. 1051.

Sutherland, D., Radosevich, D., Gruessner, A., Beilman, G., Dunn, T., Balamurugan, A. et al. (2009b). Islet autotransplant (IAT) outcomes after total pancreatectomy (TP) in the modern era. *Xenotransplantation,* Vol. 16, Issue 5, pp. 292-293.

Sutherland, D. E. R., Gruessner, A., Hering, B. J., & Gruessner, R. (2011a). Pancreas and Islet Cell Transplantation. In: *Pediatric Surgery 7th Edition,* A.Coran (Ed.). (in press).

Sutherland, D. E. R., Beilman, G., Dunn, T., Chinnakotla, S., Vickers, S., Bellin, M. et al. (2011b). Total pancreatectomy and islet-auto transplantation for chronic pancreatitis. *J Am Coll Surg.* (in press).

Sutton R, Gray DW, Burnett M, & et al. (1989). Metabolic function of intraportal and intrasplenic islet autografts in cynomolgus monkeys. *Diabetes,* Vol. 38, Suppl 1, pp. 182-184.

Sutton, J., Schmulewitz, N., Sussman, J., Smith, M., Kurland, J., Brunner, J. et al. (2010). Total pancreatectomy and islet cell autotransplantation as a means of treating patients with genetically linked pancreatitis. *Surgery,* Vol. 148, Issue 4, pp. 676-685.

Takita, M., Naziruddin, B., Matsumoto, S., Noguchi, H., Shimoda, M., Chujo, D. et al. (2010). Variables associated with islet yield in autologous islet cell transplantation for chronic pancreatitis. *Proc (Bayl Univ Med Cent),* Vol. 23, Issue 2, pp. 115-120.

Takita, M., Matsumoto, S., Qin, H., Noguchi, H., Shimoda, M., Chujo, D. et al. (2011a). Secretory Unit of Islet Transplant Objects (SUITO) Index can predict severity of hypoglycemic episodes in clinical islet cell transplantation. *Cell Transplant,* (in press).

Takita, M., Naziruddin, B., Matsumoto, S., Noguchi, H., Shimoda, M., Chujo, D. et al. (2011b). Implication of pancreatic image findings in total pancreatectomy with islet autotransplantation for chronic pancreatitis. *Pancreas*, Vol. 40, Issue 1, pp. 103-108.

Takita, M., Naziruddin, B., Matsumoto, S., Noguchi, H., Shimoda, M., Chujo, D. et al. (2011c). Body mass index reflects islet isolation outcome in islet autotransplantation for patients with chronic pancreatitis. *Cell Trans.* Vol. 20, Issue 2, pp. 313-322.

Talamini, G., Bassi, C., Falconi, M., & et al (1999). Alcohol and smoking at risk factors in chronic pancreatitis and pancreatic cancer. *Dig Dis Sci,* Vol. 44, pp. 1303-1311.

Teuscher, A. U., Kendall, D. M., Smets, Y. F. C., Leone, J. P., Sutherland, D. E. R., & Robertson, R. P. (1998). Successful islet autotransplantation in humans: Functional insulin secretory reserve as an estimate of surviving islet cell mass. *Diabetes,* Vol. 47, pp. 324-330.

Toledo-Pereyra LH, Rowlett AL, Cain W, & et al. (1984). Hepatic infarction following intraportal islet cell autotransplantation after near-total pancreatectomy. *Transplantation,* Vol. 38, Issue 1, pp. 88-89.

Traverso, L. W., Abou-Zamzam, A., & Longmire, P. (1981). Human Pancreatic Cell Autotransplantation Following Total Pancreatectomy. *Ann Surg* , Vol. 193, Issue 2, pp. 191-195.

Valente, U., Fontana, I., Arcuri, G., Costigliolo, G., Dardano, M., Pasqualini, M. et al. (1986). Critical evaluation of clinical and metabolic parameters in 27 cases of islet and segmental pancreas autotransplantation. *Transplant Proc,* Vol. 28, Issue 6, pp. 1825-1826.

Vargas F, Julian JF, Llamazares JF, & et al. (2001). Engraftment of islets obtained by collagenase and liberase in diabetic rats: a comparative study. *Pancreas,* Vol. 23, pp. 406-413.

Vega-Peralta, J., Attam, R., Arain, A., Mallery, S., Radosevich, D., Khamis, F. et al. (2011a). Correlation of EUS with Histopathology in 50 Patients Undergoing Total Pancreatectomy (TP) with Islet Autotransplantion (IAT) for Minimal Change Chronic Pancreatitis (MCCP). *GastroIntestinal Endoscopy,* Vol. 73, Issue 4S, AB324.

Vega-Peralta, J., Manivel, J., Attam, R., Arain, M., Mallery, J., Radosevich, D. et al. (2011b). Accuracy of EUS for diagnosis of minimal change chronic pancreatitis (MCCP): Correlation with histopathology in 50 patients undergoing total pancreatectomy (TP) with islet autotransplantion (IAT). *Pancreas,* (in press).

Wahoff, D. C., Hower, C., Sutherland, D. E. R., Leone, J. P., & Gores, P. F. (1994a). The peritoneal cavity: An alternative site for clinical islet transplantation? *Transplant.Proc.,* Vol. *26,* Issue *6,* pp. 3297-3298.

Wahoff, D. C., Sutherland, D. E. R., Hower, C., Lloveras, J. J., & Gores, P. F. (1994b). Free intraperitoneal islet autografts in pancreatectomized dogs - Impact of islet purity and posttransplantation exogenous insulin. *Surgery,* Issue 116, pp. 742-750.

Wahoff, D., Papalois, B., Najarian, J., & et.al. (1995a). Autologous islet transplantation to prevent diabetes after pancreatic resection. *Ann Surg,* Vol. 222, pp. 562-579.

Wahoff, D. C., Papalois, B., Najarian, J. S., Nelson, L. A., Dunn, D. L., Farney, A. C. et al. (1995b). Clinical islet autotransplantation after pancreatectomy: Determinants of success and implications for allotransplantation. *Transplant.Proc.,* Vol. 27, Issue 6, p. 3161.

Wahoff, D. C., Leone, J. P., Farney, A. C., Teuscher, A. U., & Sutherland, D. E. R. (1995c). Pregnancy after total pancreatectomy and autologous islet transplantation. *Surgery,*Vol. 117, pp. 353-354.

Wahoff, D., Papalois, B., Najarian, J., & et.al. (1996). Islet autotransplantation after total pancreatectomy in a child. *J Pediatr Surg,* Vol. 31, pp. 132-136.

Walsh TJ, Eggleston JC, & Cameron JL. (1982). Portal hypertension, hepatic infarction, and liver failure complicating pancreatic islet autotransplantation. *Surgery,* Vol. 91, pp. 485-487.

Walsh, T. N., Rode, J., Theis, B. A., & Russell, R. C. (1992). Minimal change chronic pancreatitis. *Gut,* Vol. *33,* pp. 1566-1571.

Warnock, G. L., Rajotte, R. V., & Procyshyn, A. W. (1983). Normoglycemia after reflux of islet-containing pancreatic fragments into the splenic vascular bed in dogs. *Diabetes,* Vol. 32, Issue 5, pp. 452-459.

Warshaw, A. L., Banks, P. A., & Fernandez-Del, C. C. (1998). AGA technical review: treatment of pain in chronic pancreatitis. *Gastroenterology,* Vol. 115, pp. 765-776.

Watkins, J., Krebs, A., & Rossi, R. (2003). Pancreatic autotransplantation in chronic pancreatitis. *World J Surg,* Vol. 27, Issue 11, pp. 1235-1240.

Webb, M., Illouz, S., Pollard, C., Gregory, R., Mayberry, J., Tordoff, S. et al. (2008). Islet auto transplantation following total pancreatectomy: a long-term assessment of graft function. *Pancreas,* Vol. 37, Issue 3, pp. 282-287.

Whitcomb, D. C. (2000). Genetic predisposition to acute and chronic pancreatitis. *Med Clin North Am,* Vol. *84,* pp. 531-547.

White SA, Dennison AR, Swift SM, & et al. (1998). Intraportal and splenic human islet autotransplantation combined with total pancreatectomy. *Transplant.Proc.* Vol. 30, Issue 2, pp. 312-313.

White SA, Robertson GS, London NJ, & Dennison AR. (2000a). Human islet autotransplantation to prevent diabetes after pancreas resection. *Dig Surg,* Vol. 17, Issue 5, pp. 439-450.

White SA, London NJ, Johnson PR, & et al. (2000b). The risks of total pancreatectomy and splenic islet autotransplantation. *Cell Trans.,* Vol 9, Issue 1, pp. 19-24.

White SA, Davies JE, Pollard C, & et al. (2001). Pancreas resection and islet autotransplantation for end-stage chronic pancreatitis. *Ann Surg,* Vol. 233, Issue 3, pp. 423-431.

Wilcox, C. M. & Varadarajulu, S. (2006). Endoscopic therapy for chronic pancreatitis: and evidence-based review. *Curr Gastroentrol Rep,* Vol. *8,*pp. 104-110.

Wilhelm, J. J., Bellin, M. D., Balamurugan, A. N., Beilman, G. J., Dunn, T. B., Radosevich, D. et al. (2011). A Proposed Threshold for Dispersed-Pancreatic-Tissue-Volume (TV) Infused During Intraportal- Islet-Autotransplantation (IAT) after Total-Pancreatectomy(TP) to Treat Chronic-Pancreatitis(CP). *Pancreas,* (in press).

Witt, H., Apte M.V., Keim, V., & et al (2011). Chronic pancreatitis: challenges and advances in pathogensis, genetics, diagnosis, and therapy. *Gastroenterology,* Vol. *132,* pp. 1557-1573.